Keto For Women Over 50

A Complete Beginner's Guide for Women Over 50 to Loose Weight and Heal Your Body Through Keto Diet

Jenni Treesong

Table of Contents

INTRODUCTION 1

What Is the Ketogenic Diet? 3

    Basic of Low-Carb Diet 4

Low-Carb Diet Benefits for Women 7

Benefits of keto for women over 50. 9

Main Differences For Women In Keto Diet. 16

What To Eat/Avoid On A Low-Carb Diet. 21

In First Week, What To Expect. 24

Sample Low-Carb Meal Plan. 26

Myths Of The Keto Diet. 28

How to Get Started with Keto For Women Over 50. ... 38

Ketogenic Diet Tips For Women Over 50 47

Keto Diet Recipes 64

Breakfast 64

    Sheet Pan Eggs 64

    Paleo Breakfast Pizza 66

    Gluten Free Bacon and Egg Muffins 69

    Creamy Cauliflower and Ground Beef Skillet 71

Coconut Flour Porridge 74

Liver Sausage and Eggs 76

Strawberry Avocado Keto Smoothie with Almond Milk 78

Ground Beef, Eggs and Avocado Breakfast Bowl 80

Guacamole Deviled Eggs 82

Steak and Eggs 84

Keto Breakfast Burger with Avocado Buns 86

Breakfast BLT Salad 89

Snacks 91

Sugar Free Low Carb Keto Avocado Brownies 91

3 Ingredient Keto Peanut Butter Cookies 94

Sugar Free Low Carb Keto Avocado Brownies 96

Peanut Butter Power Granola 99

Lemon Strawberry Cheesecake Treats 101

Classic Chocolate Cake Donuts 103

Pistachio toffee cups 106

Keto Coconut Mocha Doughnuts 109

Keto Cinnamon Roll Biscotti 111

Avocado Popsicle with Coconut & Lime 115

Classic Blueberry Scones 117

Salad And Side Dish 120

Peanut Butter & Jam Cups 120

Homemade Caramel Frappuccino 123

Keto Broccoli Salad with Cheese and Bacon 125

Keto Carrot Cake 127

Keto Lemon Bars 130

Baked Cauliflower Casserole with Goat Cheese 132

Mexican Cauliflower "Rice" 135

Cheddar Bacon Cauliflower Potato Salad 137

Low Carb Macaroni Salad 139

Cheesy Cauliflower alla Vodka Casserole 141

Lunch And Dinner 143

Loaded Chicken Salad 143

Crack Slaw Egg Roll in a Bowl 147

Sesame Salmon w. Baby Bok Choy & Mushrooms. 149

Low Carb Keto Chili 151

Lemon Balsamic Chicken 153

Salmon Gremolata with Roasted Vegetables 156

Low Carb Beef Stir Fry 159

BBQ Pulled Beef Sando 161

Cauliflower Mac and Cheese Recipe & Keto Cheese Sauce 164

Keto Meatloaf 167

Caprese Tuna Salad Stuffed Tomatoes 170

Any Time Keto Recipes 172

Keto Cream Cheese Bread 172

Parmesan & Tomato Keto Bread Buns 176

15-Minute Gluten Free, Low Carb & Keto Tortillas 180

Cheddar Garlic Fathead Rolls 184

Gluten Free, Paleo & Keto Bread............................ 187

Keto Mini Bread Loaves... 193

Collagen Keto Bread.. 196

Coconut Flour Pizza Crust...................................... 199

Gluten Free, Paleo & Keto Drop Biscuits 203

Low Carb Bagels-Gluten Free Onion Sesame.......... 207

Cranberry Jalapeño "Cornbread" Muffins............... 209

Paleo Chocolate Zucchini Bread 212

Garlic, Dill & Cheddar Keto Bread 217

Cauliflower Bread Recipe with Garlic & Herbs....... 221

Keto Bagel Recipe.. 225

Keto Pull Apart Clover Rolls................................... 228

Keto Flax Seed Bread 231

3 Minute Low Carb Biscuits 233

Coconut Flour Psyllium Husk Bread - Paleo........... 235

Homemade Nut and Seed Paleo Bread 238

Low Carb Pumpkin Bread 241

Cheesy Skillet Bread 244

Turmeric Cauliflower Buns 247

Buttery Low Carb Flatbread.................................... 251

Paleo Gluten-Free Low Carb English Muffin.......... 254

Cauliflower Tortillas 257

Keto Fiber Bread Rolls Recipe 260

Low Carb Gluten Free Cranberry Bread 263

Low Carb Focaccia Bread 266

Cinnamon Raisin Swirl Bread 269

Keto Low Carb Buns with Psyllium Husk 273

3 Ingredient Paleo Naan (Indian bread) 277

Ultimate Dairy-Free Keto Bread 280

Best Keto Bread Recipe 283

Keto + Low Carb Cornbread Muffins 286

Keto Flax Seed Bread 290

3 Minute Low Carb Biscuits 292

Coconut Flour Psyllium Husk Bread - Paleo 294

Homemade Nut and Seed Paleo Bread 297

Low Carb Pumpkin Bread 300

Cheesy Skillet Bread 303

Turmeric Cauliflower Buns 306

Buttery Low Carb Flatbread 310

Paleo Gluten-Free Low Carb English Muffin 313

Cauliflower Tortillas 316

Keto Fiber Bread Rolls Recipe 319

CONCLUSION 322

INTRODUCTION

Looking for a diet that encourages rapid weight loss? Women's keto diet ranks 13th best out of 40 diets in this area. It's also beneficial in middle-aged women with signs of menopause and overall health. Continue reading to learn more about your weight-loss and health benefits.

Many women in postmenopause (over 50) tend to gain weight. It's a decline in sex hormones in large measure. For men the same thing happens when their testosterone is declining.

One major benefit of ketogenic diets is that the insulin levels in the body are really lower. This is largely due to their low carbohydrate content, but also due to a generally reduced caloric intake in these diets by people.

You address a root problem in post-menopausal women and an obesity mechanism by taking a ketogenic diet. You help address the issue of insulin resistance in the body by lowering the insulin levels in the body. Regarding weight this should be improving significantly.

The ketogenic diet is not some new, untested "fad." It was first commonly used to treat epileptic children starting in the early 1900's. It has been discovered in study after study to beat other diets in weight loss while helping to improve metabolic markers associated with heart disease and body inflammation in the body.

Jenni Treesong

What Is the Ketogenic Diet?

The keto diet plan has been in existence for almost 100 years. It has diagnosed children successfully with drug-resistant epilepsy. In the 1970s Dr. Atkins launched his very-low-carbohydrate diet in his cardiology clinics for weight loss. He figured out that, they held it off when they lost weight. By mistake Atkins is Keto... the big difference is that protein consumption should be somewhat reduced.

A normal diet which has a moderate to high intake of carb causes the body to use glucose as its source of fuel. Keto diet theory is that eating low carb foods and not consuming too much protein will help your body not rely on energy for glucose but rather on ketones.

Basic of Low-Carb Diet

There is no one-size-fits-all low-carb diet guide, but most plans launch off on a very low-carb diet schedule, adding carbohydrates gradually and slowly once weight is lost. According to the Mayo Clinic, low-carb diets typically start by limiting carbohydrates down to 20 to 60 grams per day. Many carbohydrates consumed in low-carb diet come from vegetables such as leafy greens or cauliflower.

Most low carb diets gradually reintroduce carbs into the meal plan after people lose weight. According to Cleveland Clinic, carb cycling is a popular way for many people to reintegrate carbs into their diet. That involves organizing your weekly carb consumption based on your more or less active days. You eat meals with a slightly higher carb count on days you're more involved, thus you go back to low carb on more sedentary days.

A very successful weight loss plan is ketogenic diet. To burn fat instead of glucose it uses high fat and low carbohydrate ingredients. Many people are familiar with the Atkins diet but the keto plan further restricts carbs.

Since we're surrounded by fast food restaurants and packaged meals, avoiding carb-rich foods can be a challenge, but proper planning will help.

Prepare meals and snacks at least a week in advance, so you don't get stuck with just high carb meal choices. Study keto recipes; you can choose from quite a few good ones. Plunge into the keto lifestyle, find your favorite recipes and stick to them.

A couple of items are staples of a keto diet. Make sure those items are on hand:.

Eggs-Used in omelets, quiches (yes, heavy cream is legal on keto!), hard-boiled as a snack, low-carbon pizza crust, and more; if you like eggs, you're very likely to succeed on this Bacon diet–do I need a reason? Breakfast, salad garnish, burger topper, BLT's (no toast, of course; try a BLT in a cup, tossed in mayo) Cream cheese— hundreds of recipes, pizza crusts, main dishes, desserts Shredded cheese — Sprinkle over taco meat in a bowl, turned into microwave tortilla chips, salad toppers, low-carb pizza and enchiladas Plenty of roman and spinach — fill up on green veggies; have plenty at your fingers; Or crumble and cook with taco seasoning and use in provolone cheese taco shells; throw in a lettuce dish, avocado, cheese, sour cream for tortilla-less taco salad Almonds (plain or flavored)-these are a delicious and healthy snack; but be sure to count them as you eat, because the carbs add up. Habanero, mango, salt and vinegar and more flavours.

Jenni Treesong

Low-Carb Diet Benefits for Women.

According to the (AARP) American Association of Retired Persons, both low-carb and low-fat diets can be effective for weight loss. The low-carb diet, however, does have some additional health benefits worth considering. The above research tested the impact of low-carb and low-fat diets on knee pain in adults with osteoarthritis, which affects many people. Researchers shown that the low-carb diet was more effective in reducing knee pain after assigning participants to either low-carbon or low-fat diets. The low-carb diet can offer an alternative to opioids that relieve pain.

In addition, low-carb diets may help to improve the levels of HDL (good) cholesterol and triglycerides more effectively than more carb-heavy diets, the Mayo Clinic reports. This is may probably due in part to the low-carb diet nature — lots of lean protein, healthy fats, and unprocessed carbs — so food choices are typically healthier than the standard American diet.

Low-carb diets today have taken several popular forms including the keto diet, the paleo diet, and the Mediterranean diet. Whereas each of these options has its own complexities, all of them are based on lowering the intake of carbohydrate while increasing healthy fat.

Benefits of keto for women over 50.

Keto is mostly seen as a diet for weight loss. Nevertheless, low-carb keto diets offer women in their 50s some other significant benefits.

These advantages include:

Improved Blood Lipid Profile.

Most females experience increased triglyceride and "poor" LDL cholesterol levels in their 50s.

While high in fat, low carb diets have been shown to reduce triglycerides and LDL cholesterol while increasing the "healthy" HDL cholesterol levels.

Both improvements are related to improved cardiovascular health and lower heart disease risk

Reduced Body Fat.

Some of the diets promise weight loss but that weight is mostly water in many cases. Keto increases the burning of fat and achieves better results than most other diets. Keto also targets abdominal fat preferentially, properly called visceral fat Abdominal fat tends to increase over 50 in women. That raises the risk of heart disease, heart arrest and stroke. The accumulation of abdominal fat is due in large part to the increases in hormone associated with menopause.

Reduced Inflammation.

The process of aging can be difficult on your body. In their 50s, menopausal women experience knee and hip pain, as well as headaches and other forms of non-specific pain.

Keto is a high-fat diet and it is very useful to calm inflammation with some fats. Good anti-inflammatory fats to be part of your keto diet include:.

- ❖ Olive oil.
- ❖ Oily fish, for example sardines, tuna, and salmon.
- ❖ Avocados and avocado oil.
- ❖ Walnuts.

Foods such as refined carbs, sugar, and processed foods are all associated with increased inflammation, by contrast. These foods aren't part of the keto diet.

Blood Pressure Reduced

Women tend to have less blood pressure than men. When you enter your 50s, though, that can change, and menopause begins to take hold.

High blood pressure is associated with a host of serious health issues, including kidney disease, stroke and heart disease. The low-carb keto diet has been proven to help decrease blood pressure.

Insulin Sensitivity Increased.

Carbs are digested, and glucose is converted. Your body produces the hormone insulin when you eat carbs, to ferry the glucose into your liver and muscles. With age, though, the sensitivity of your body to insulin decreases, and that means that glucose is more likely to be converted into and stored as fat, resulting in weight gain.

The low carb diets increasing the sensitivity to insulin. Which means the few carbs which you eat will not turn into fat. The increased sensitivity to insulin also helps to regulate the blood glucose levels. Low blood glucose levels are inextricably linked to better general health and a decreased risk of developing type 2 diabetes.

Less Muscle Loss.

Women in their fifties tend to lose muscle faster than those in their twenties, thirties and forties. Loss of muscle decreases the metabolic rate, contributing to weight gain and making it more difficult to lose weight.

Losing muscle will also have an effect on your strength, making everyday activities more difficult and tiring.

Ketogenic diet involves eating moderate protein amounts, and protein is vital for perseverance of the muscles. Protein contains amino acids, and the building blocks of muscle tissue are amino acids.

Enhanced Brain Function.

Menopausal women often experience things like loss of memory, mood swings and concentration difficulties. They may even suffer from anxiety and depression. This is because estrogen levels, the primary female sex hormone, decline during menopause, affecting the amount of glucose that reaches your brain.

The Keto diet provides an alternative source of fuel for your brain; ketones. Your brain works best on ketones, and problems like mood swings and memory loss on a low-carb diet are far less common.

The keto diet is also related to a reduced risk of many neurological conditions, including Alzheimer's and Parkinson's disease, both of which are more prevalent in individuals over 50 years old.

Increased Bone Mass.

Older women are vulnerable to bone loss which can become osteoporosis if left unchecked. This is a medical condition characterized by fracture-prone, weak bones.

Keto eliminates nutrients which can interfere with the absorption of calcium. Keto can also help improve both bone health and density combined with lots of leafy green vegetables that are naturally high in calcium.

It's easy to see that keto can be very beneficial to women in their 50s–both for weight loss and health enhancement.

Going on keto diet means cutting out many of the unhealthy foods we know, and replacing them with foods that are high in beneficial nutrients.

Keto, in short, is not just a diet for people overweight; it is a diet for anyone who wish to live a longer, healthier life!

Main Differences For Women In Keto Diet.

The bodies of women are unique in many aspects. However, as with any strategy to lose weight, there is no one-size-fits-all diet. There are many ketogenic diet strategies but most women require changes to fulfill their dietary needs.

The keto diet is among women's best diets for rapid weight loss. It is however restrictive when it comes to food choices. You may become nutrient deficient. Check with your doctor to see if you need a multi-vitamin or any other supplement before you start.

Women face complications such as menopause, imbalances in the hormones, anemia and osteoporosis. It is important to draw up a diet plan which evolves to meet the changing nutritional needs of a woman. Choosing foods which are rich in calcium, iron, magnesium, vitamin D and vitamin B9 (folate) will prevent any dietary deficiencies.

What works best for one woman might not be the best for another. Having your dietary choices for your individual nutritional needs is important. These may include enhancing your energy, fighting stress, reducing symptoms of PMS or alleviating menopause symptoms. Following a daily meal plan will help you stay safe and productive every step of your life.

Who is a suitable candidate?

A lot of women benefit from taking a keto diet. For weight loss, most people turn to it but it can also improve a woman's overall health. Women who experience any of the conditions below can see changes.

- ❖ Inactivity.
- ❖ Polycystic Ovarian Syndrome.
- ❖ Obesity.

- ❖ Menopause.
- ❖ Epilepsy.
- ❖ Diabetes Diabetes
- ❖ Cardiovascular Illness.

Women's low carb, high fat diet helps to increase satiety and reduce appetite. Consuming products like Fat Fit Go which contain the right amount of nutrients and which taste great compliance boost. When you are on the go, you can take them to anywhere you travel as a healthy snack.

Is the Keto Diet Safe? Or do I need to consult with my doctor?

Adopting the keto diet without a doctor visit is healthy for most females. But there are certain cases a doctor may administer the diet. Including:.

- ❖ Breastfeeding.
- ❖ Adjustment of diabetes medications.
- ❖ Blood pressure adjustment medications.
- ❖ Pregnancy.

Keto for women over 50 is a safe and useful weight loss tool if followed by a doctor. Medical support is an additional precaution for ensuring your nutritional success. Monitoring blood pressure and glucose levels increases your sense of wellbeing as well as your mood.

To Keto or Not To Keto?

Ever thinking about adopting the keto diet? Research studies indicate that in other health disorders a low carb diet for women has a sound scientific basis for successful weight loss and progress.

Have you started a keto diet but initially got discouraged by exhaustion and low levels of energy? The body turns from using glucose to ketones as its principal source of energy. The first few weeks can be tough because the body adjusts.

A few simple tricks will lighten the side effects. The success of this diet depends on hydration with water or herbal tea. Dehydration can make you feel lightheaded and slow. A regular sleep and exercise routine also helps to reduce unwanted side effects by offering tried and true advice. + Electrolytes.

Can you put your keto diet to work? The response is a big, resounding yes! It'll take you some time to plan and prepare meals before you feel confident about your food choices. But once you learn the foods that you can choose to satisfy, it becomes second nature.

Jenni Treesong

What To Eat/Avoid On A Low-Carb Diet.

You'll eat more carb-free proteins including beef, pork, chicken, turkey, eggs and seafood to keep the carbs low. Cheese is as well rich in protein but most varieties have about one gram per ounce of carbohydrates.

According to the University of California San Francisco Medical Center, fiber is important for women in their 40s, however, as it prevents blood sugar levels from spiking too quickly. A low-carb diet makes getting the recommended 25 grams a day difficult for you, which is why it is necessary to include plenty of non-starchy veggies on your plan.

This includes sprouts of alfalfa, asparagus, spinach, choy bok, kale, broccoli, cauliflower, mushrooms, cucumbers, lettuce, and oignons. According to Yale Medicine, such vegetables each have five grams of net carbs or less per serving. Because they don't spike your blood sugar, they're not included in the "net carb" count, which refers to the carb content in foods after subtracting the fibre.

Often, fruits are high in fibre, but many are too high in carbs to match a low-carb strategy. Pumpkin, olives, and avocados each have fewer than 5 grams of net carbs per serving, however.

Soy foods, including tempeh, tofu and edamame, are also low in net carbs, with three to six grams per serving, and serve as an alternative meat source for protein. While some soy foods are packed with fibre, vitamins, and minerals, according to Harvard Health Publishing, stay away from soy isoflavone supplements and foods that contain soy protein isolate.

Eventually, add carb-free fats such as olive oil, ghee, or avocado oil to your meals. Beware of salad dressings, since many of them contain secret sugars. And think about making your own low-carb dressing!

Avoid:

- ❖ Starchy vegetables (winter squash and potatoes)
- ❖ High carb fruits like bananas and apples.
- ❖ Products which have sugar.
- ❖ Cereal.
- ❖ Grains such as maize, wheat, and rice.

The trick is not to get frustrated here. You'll build your own eating style that works for you as you learn more about the ins and outs of the diet. Planning your meals in advance will take away much of the pressure that surrounds what to eat.

Finding a support group nearby or an online group where you can have answers to questions and see the successes of others can help. Fellow dieters inspiration will give you encouragement when you struggle.

In First Week, What To Expect.

In the first weeks of the ketogenic diet the weight loss is uncertain. The calorie needs change every day. And the amount you eat, on any given day, will not be the same. That means the results of weight loss will not follow a set pattern.

There are times you don't lose weight. And then you could lose 4-5 pounds in the next week. The key to weight loss in the long term is discipline, being consistent with your plan and staying positive through the challenges.

Losing an average of 1 (one) to 2 (two) pounds per week is an acceptable weight loss goal. Keep up what you are doing once you reach this goal. If you are on a plateau or stop losing weight, you may need to adjust to your diet.

Another choice to start weight-loss again is intermittent fasting. Fasting will jump-start your body for a specified amount of time to consume all its glucose reserves and get you back into ketoses.

Finally, raising your life's tension will go a long way towards keeping ketosis going. Yoga, meditation on mindfulness and deep-breathing exercises are excellent techniques for relaxation.

Sample Low-Carb Meal Plan.

If you are set on 30 grams of carbs a day, you could have a crustless frittata made with eggs, Swiss cheese, sliced asparagus and onions for breakfast; serve it with bacon or cooked ham. Or try two low-carb pancakes made from a baking mix of low-carb almond flour.

You may choose to stir-fried lean chicken breast with broccoli, bok choy, mung bean sprouts, sesame oil and soy sauce for lunch. Mixed greens topped with chopped steak, sliced boiled eggs, cucumbers, crumbled bacon, and an olive oil dressing may also be considered.

Complete the day with roasted Brussels sprouts and turnips, broiled salmon. A bunless burger with cheddar cheese, lettuce and tomato is a good dinner too. Serve with fresh green beans sauteed in garlic and olive oil.

Avocado, hard-boiled eggs, celery sticks, olives or sliced cucumbers are among the low-carb snack options. Although deli meats are "allowed" to a low-carb diet, according to the University of Virginia UVA Cancer Center, they also contain harmful ingredients, such as nitrates. Wisely choose your deli meats.

If you need to spare a few carbohydrates, put in a couple of fibre-rich nuts every once in a while. An ounce of pecans, hazelnuts, or almonds each produce one to three grams of net carbs. But be mindful of the calorie count, if you're in it for weight loss. Nuts are nutritious but calorie-dense snacks so be sure to eat the right portion.

Myths Of The Keto Diet.

Keto Is High in Protein.

Unlike what you might have heard (or what's tagged on Instagram with #keto), protein isn't the focus of the keto diet— and too much of it can actually throw off track. The body will turn protein into glucose, which it can then use for fuel rather than fat, taking you out of the fat-burning environment you are striving to achieve.

Although protein will not be the star of your plate, a keto diet can still satisfy your needs. Many people require between 0.8 and 1 gram of protein per kg of body weight, which is just around 55 gs per day for someone weighing 150 pounds, says dietitian Kristen Mancinelli, M.S., R.D.N., who specializes in low carb diets. Getting there requires just three ounces of salmon (20 grams), three ounces of chicken (28 grams), and either an ounce of almonds or an egg (6 grams each).

Low-Carb And Keto Are Fundamentally The Same.

Although a keto diet is of course low-carb, a low-carb diet is not necessarily keto, Mancinelli says. About 100 grams of carbs a day would be considered low carb for most people. On keto, that intake needs to be significantly lower, around 20 to 30 grams a day — although people who are very active and have a lot of lean body mass may be able to handle a bit more. Eat just too many grams of carbs and change the body right back to burning sugar for food, she says.

Keto Isn't Long-Term Sustainability

It's true, the rigid nature of keto isn't for everyone, but people who enjoy structure and routine can really do well in the long-term diet, Jadin says. "A lot of people have adopted a keto diet for years," she says. The key to making keto work is to think of it as a lifestyle and not just a' diet'—and many people are so inspired by weight loss and health benefits the after-keto experience that they are able to make it a permanent lifestyle, Jadin says.

Going keto for good may still sound daunting, but a growing body of research indicates certain benefits to metabolic and cognitive health may be beneficial.

Pre-planning meals and bringing keto-friendly snacks such as nuts, seeds, cheese sticks and hard-boiled eggs will help you stay on board with long-term keto.

On Keto You Don't Eat Veggies.

One big misconception about keto is that there's no space on your plate for vegetables, mostly because they contain too many carbohydrates. Yet plant-based foods— and the vitamins, minerals, and fiber that they provide — are essential to a healthy keto diet, Jadin advises.

True, you're going to want to steer clear of starchy vegetables like potatoes and corn that quickly rack up the carbs; but you can (and should) still load on non-starchy vegetables— especially fiber-rich leafy vegetables. For example, spinach, arugula, and broccoli all contain fewer than two grans of net carbs per serving.

Start with your fat source when preparing your meals and then add a non-starchy veggie, Jadin says. You may have a vegetable omelet for breakfast; for lunch and dinner, help yourself with a serve of greens sautéed in butter.

They Can Eat Any Fat Type.

The keto diet might seem like a free-for-all dietary fat (how else should you get 90 per cent of your total daily calories from bacon-free fat?), but experts stress that a keto diet does not give you the green light to fill up with saturated sources.

According to the American College of Nutrition's Paper, substituting saturated fat (bacon, sausages, ham, etc.) with unsaturated fat (walnuts, flax seeds, shrimp, etc.) is more effective in reducing cardiovascular disease risk than simply reducing total fat intake. Meanwhile, work ties eating processed meats (such as bacon) to increasing cancer risks.

"When you put a Mediterranean flair on it, maximize your ketogenic lifestyle," says Roehl. "Concentrate on getting the most of your calories from the high-quality extra virgin olive oil, nuts and seeds, and fatty fish."

As mentioned earlier, ketosis is when your body is in optimum "fat burning" mode, and that can only happen if your body uses fat stores for energy and ketone output. But that is not to be confused with ketoacidosis, says Jim White, R.D.N., owner of Virginia Beach's Jim White Fitness and Nutrition Studios. Ketoacidosis is a life-threatening disease in which the blood of the body is highly acidic, and is seen most often in people with diabetes.

Nevertheless, ketoacidosis can occur in people adopting a ketogenic diet, because the disorder is caused by extremely high levels of ketones, according to a 2017 study published in the Strength and Conditioning Journal. Ketoacidosis signs include pain in the abdomen, fatigue, hunger, shortness of breath, nausea, and blurred vision. This brings us to the following myth... Ketosis side effects.

There are many amazing benefits with taking a low-carb ketogenic diet, such as weight loss, reduced cravings, and possibly reducing the risk of disease. That being said, it's also good to talk about possible side effects of keto diet so you know well what to expect when you begin this new journey of health.

It Could Boost Levels In Your A1C.

Diabetes? According to a recent study of ketogenic diets, improved blood sugar control could help control the A1C levels, and even reduce the insulin requirement. (Just don't go off your medicines without first talking to your doctor!) An important caveat? Eating keto also increases the risk of diabetic ketoacidosis— a life-threatening disease in which fat breaks down too quickly and causes the blood to acidise. It's a lot more common in people with type 1 diabetes, but if you have T2D and eat keto, talk to your doctor about what to do to reduce your risk.

Problems With Sleeping.

For dysfunction of the HPA axis you are likely to experience a sleep disturbance. This is because melatonin is antagonistic to cortisol (meaning it is in opposition to its function). When thrown off the HPA axis, levels of cortisol begin to fluctuate and interfere with melatonin release occurring at nighttime.

To briefly review hypoglycemia stimulates cortisol release. Cortisol signalling the release of accumulated glucose from the liver and muscle tissue in the body, called glycogen. Cortisol is a stimulating hormone that can cause sleep disruption if that response occurs at night. It leads either to insomnia or to very poor sleep quality.

Although this response to cortisol is helpful in emergencies, during keto-adaptation and especially at night you want to give it a try and minimize it as much as you can.

Dizziness & Drowsiness.

If you are hypoglycemic while not completely keto-adapted, you essentially have an energy deficit inside the body. This is a short-term adaptation which can result in a number of keto side effects.

You will probably feel dizzy and drowsy during this period, due to a general lack of energy. You may feel particularly dizzy when you are standing due to dysregulation of blood pressure and inappropriate response of cortisol (dysregulation of the HPA axis which we will address shortly).

Strength & Physical Performance Reduced.

During keto-adaptation, your body learns to use a completely new source of fuel that it wasn't forced to use before. The muscles contain lots of mitochondria (along with the brain) that must now learn to use ketones as a source of energy for energy production.

During this time, you will likely feel a significant decrease in strength and ability to exert physical energy as one of the side effects of short-term keto. Fortunately, once you have adapted, you should see drastic improvements in these areas that are even greater than when you have adapted to sugar!

You May Experience Less Brain Fog.

It's no secret that carbs— particularly refined ones such as sugar, white bread and white pasta— Spike up and dip your blood sugar. Therefore it makes sense to eat less of them can help keep things nice and even. This can lead to more stable energy for healthy people, less brain fog and less sugar cravings, says Mancinelli.

You're Likely Feeling Extra Thirsty.

Don't be surprised if you get parched while on the ketogenic diet. Mancinelli advises that excreting all that extra water will likely cause a spike in thirst— so make it a point to drink. There's no recommendation for how much water you should have on a keto diet, hard and quick. In general, however, aim to drink enough so your urine is either clear or pale yellow.

How to Get Started with Keto For Women Over 50.

While keto is a straightforward diet, making the transition from a high carb diet to eating 50 grams or less of carbs per day isn't always easy.

By following these guidelines make your transition into low carb keto diet easier.

Understand That Going Keto Is Not Always Easy For The First Two Weeks-Especially For The First Two Weeks.

It takes your body time to use all of its onboard carb reserves, and instead make the move to use ketones for energy.

During this time, some people experience unpleasant side effects which are commonly called keto flu.

Although keto flu isn't dangerous and it certainly doesn't catch, you can feel unwell before your body reaches ketosis in full.

Symptoms typical to keto flu include:.

- ❖ Headaches.
- ❖ Nausea.
- ❖ Constipation.
- ❖ Increased urination.
- ❖ Tiredness.
- ❖ Mood swings.
- ❖ Cravings.
- ❖ Insomnia.
- ❖ Fruity-smelling breath.

The great news is that these signs show your body is beginning to move from using carbs to using ketones for energy. You are well on the way to becoming a tool that burns fat. Your symptoms will soon disappear, and they will completely pass over within 1-2 weeks.

Also, once they've passed, and you'll only experience keto flu once unless you cheat on your diet.

Clear The Unwanted Carbohydrates From Your Cupboards.

Clean your kitchen cupboards and the refrigerator of any non-keto foods just before you start your keto diet.

You may think you can overcome the temptation and not consume them, but the fact is that if you have easy access to high-carb foods, you are more likely to break your diet.

Nevertheless do not make the mistake of eating all these foods. The harder and slower the transition into ketosis is, the more carbs you eat in the lead up to keto.

Consider Using Supplements Which Are Well Selected.

Although you don't have to use keto diet supplements they can make things easier for women over 50 years of age. Good choices include: 2. Triglycerides with medium chain.

In short, the MCTs quickly and easily convert these special fats into ketones. Less ketones means increased fat burning and weight loss, less strength and less symptoms of keto flu.

The MCT supplements are made from coconut oil or palm oil. Coconut oil, however, is the cheapest, and is also the most environmentally friendly alternative. MCTs are available as oils or in simple to mix type of powder.

Exogenous Ketones.

Exogenous ketones are extraneous source ketones. Taking exogenous ketone supplements can stimulate the burning of fat, keep your mind clear, give you strength and can help reduce many of the symptoms of keto flu. Exogenous ketones can be used as tablets and as blends for beverages.

Electrolytes.

Electrolytes are minerals in your urine that are excreted and also lose as you sweat.

The keto diet increases the output of urine, and that can mean that your body starts running low on these critical substances. Signs of low electrolyte levels include muscle cramps and headaches.

Electrolyte supplements replace the minerals missing and can help prevent several of the keto flu symptoms.

Have A Planned Start Date.

Keto diet is so different from other diets that without doing your homework, you can not just jump in.

Choose a start date and let yourself read about the ins and outs of low-carb diet.

Learn about what to eat & what not to eat. Spend this time collecting any low-carb tools, such as meal plans and recipes, that might be helpful.

Also, tell your family and friends that you're "going keto" and that your diet is about to change.

Tell them to be patient and accept that in the foreseeable future, you will not be eating bread, rice, pasta, etc.

Don't Cheat Anyway!

Most diets encourage you to have days off and even cheat from time to time, by eating unhealthy foods. The keto diet is no such diet! When you cheat on keto by eating carbs, You're going to get kicked out of ketosis and have to go through another stretch of keto flu to get back on track.

A long story, don't be tempted to cheat on keto-it just isn't worth it. Alternatively, use other types of treatments to reward your positive dietary habits.

Good options such as going to the movies, buying a new fitness outfit or treating yourself to a beauty treatment or massage. High carb food treatments do not form part of a ketogenic diet.

Use An App For Food Monitoring.

Successful keto diet means the carb consumption is limited to 50 grams or less per day.

The best, if not the only way, is to use a food tracking app to do that successfully.

This includes good choices.

- ❖ My Fitness Pal,
- ❖ My Macros+,
- ❖ My Plate.

Armed with your easy-to-use macro tracker, you can fine-tune your meals to get calories, protein and fat intake right.

Treat Keto As Lifestyle Rather Than Just Diet.

When most people think of a new diet they just plan to follow it for a couple of weeks. They figure that they will suffer through it until they have lost some weight, and then they go back to their former eating way. It inevitably results in weight loss followed by weight recovery-what experts call yoyo diet.

When you view low-carb diet as a lifestyle choice, and not a short-term remedy, you will get much better results with keto. You're not only going to lose weight this way, but you're going to keep it off for good too.

Furthermore, most of the advantages mentioned in this book earlier only apply while you are dieting low in carb. You can say goodbye to things like lower blood pressure, improved cardiovascular health, reduced inflammation and improved bone health if you break your diet.

Keto is good for weight loss in your 50s, but that too can be so much more. It can have a profound and significant effect on every aspect of your wellbeing.

Don't throw away the advantages after a few weeks or months, by hitting and leaving keto. Instead, commit yourself long-term to low-carb diet. If you do you will love the results.

Jenni Treesong

Ketogenic Diet Tips For Women Over 50.

A ketogenic diet is a meal plan based on very low carbohydrates, moderate protein, and high fat.

A ketogenic diet trains the metabolism of the individual so that fatty acids or ketone bodies run off. This is called adapted fat, when the body has adapted to run off at rest of the fatty acids / ketones.

This diet program has been demonstrated to improve the response to insulin and to reduce inflammation. It leads to lower chronic disease incidence and better muscle development and fat metabolism.

With this diet plan the biggest challenge is to get into and sustain the fat adaptation condition. Here are several advanced diet tips for getting into ketosis and keeping it there.

Enhance Your Sleep.

When you sleep badly, you can increase the stress hormones and cause dysregulatory issues with blood sugar. Be sure to get up at a good time (before 11 pm) to go to sleep and sleep in a completely dark room. Depending on your stress levels, sleeping 7-9 hours each night (more stress means you need more sleep) and the amount you feel like you need to feel good and mentally alert all day.

Keep your room cool (usually suitable at 60-65 degrees) with an overhead ventilator supplying fresh air. Use a sleep mask to block out more light disrupting melatonin.

If you are extremely sensitive to sound or in a louder area, it can be extremely helpful to use ear plugs!

Practice Intermittent Fasting.

This is one of the great ways to get in and keep ketosis because you reduce calories and don't consume protein or carbs. To stop a hypoglycemic episode it is a good idea to go low-carb for at least a few days before beginning this.

Exercise Regularly.

We could talk all day about nutrition-focusing ketogenic diet tips but it's important to transfer quality. Daily, high-intensity exercise in the liver and muscle tissue helps to activate the glucose transport molecule called the GLUT-4 receptor. The GLUT-4 receptor serves to remove sugar from the blood stream and store it as glycogen in the liver and muscles. Regular exercise increases the Muscle and Liver levels of this essential protein.

This is a very important adaptation to maintain ketosis, as it will allow the individual to handle a little more carbohydrates in the diet as the body wants to store them in the muscle and liver tissue.

Large compound exercises which use multiple muscle groups have the greatest impact on the activity of GLUT-4 receptors. It involves squats, deadlifts, push-ups, overhead presses standing, and pull-ups, or pull-downs, or bent over sets.

Incorporate a regular exercise program which includes these resistance exercises as well as running sprints and low intensity exercise such as walking helps balance blood sugar and enhance the ability to get into ketosis and keep it going.

Don't overdo it just be sure. Small quantities of high intensity training are going a long way. If you overtrain your body, higher amounts of stress hormones will be secreted which will drive up blood sugar then pull you out of ketosis.

Here's a sample to support exercise program.

- ❖ Monday: 15-20 mins of Upper Body Resistance Training.
- ❖ Tuesday: 15-20 mins lower body resistance training.
- ❖ Wednesday: Walk about the block for 30 minutes.

- ❖ Thursday: 15-20 mins of Upper Body Resistance Training.
- ❖ Friday: 15-20 mins of lower body resistance training.
- ❖ Sat / Sun: Walking and recreational activities.

If you are a high-level athlete or do an intense regular exercise like Crossfit, consult with your coach or trainer who is familiar with your goal of achieving a ketosis state and modify the training based on that.

If you are struggling with a chronic illness or have stage III adrenal fatigue then I would recommend that you do no intense exercise and instead focus on stretching and breathing exercises such as yoga and tai chi and low-impact movement such as light walking or elliptical exercises.

Wisely Choose Carbs.

We all know that keto diet is a low-carb plan but in a protein shake consumes nutrient-rich carbohydrate sources such as non-starchy veggies and small amounts of low-glycemic fruits such as lemon, lime and/or a handful of berries. One of the ketogenic diet tips is regularly bringing in carbohydrates, like once a week.

Once a week, as you come out of ketosis, you raise your carbohydrates on that particular day by adding lots of grass-fed butter and cinnamon in nutrient-dense sources such as more berries in a shake or a sweet potato. Avoid the sweet potato on low carb days and keep the berries to a tiny handful at most.

Six (6) Low carb days with no more than one (1) serving of fruit (other than lemon / limes) and no starchy veggies with no more than 40 grams of net carbs (not counting fibre).

1 higher carb day with 2 portions of antioxidant rich low-glycemic fruit and 1-2 portions of starchy veggies (yam, sweet potato, pumpkin, carrot or beet) and up to 80 grams of net carbohydrates.

Boost The Motility Of Your Bowel.

Constipation is one of the biggest challenges a ketogenic diet has for men. You won't be able to stay in ketosis if you are constipated, as it drives up stress hormones and blood sugar. Constipation is often a consequence of one of the following:

- ❖ Pre-existing constipation struggles due to overgrowth of the small intestinal bacteria (SIBO) or Candida.
- ❖ Not consuming enough fibrous vegetables & fermented foods, snacks, and tonics.
- ❖ Dehydration.
- ❖ Inadequate intake of electrolytes (notably sodium, potassium, calcium and magnesium).
- ❖ Chronic stress that shuts the gastrocolic contractions down.

The ketogenic diet recommendations to fix this are to address any bacterial or yeast problems overgrowth by eating fermented foods if tolerable such as kimchi, sauerkraut, apple cider vinegar, pickles, etc. It is advised to do extra magnesium supplementation and consume a lot of clean water and to add extra sodium in pink salts. Doing a fresh green drink daily will also help to increase levels of potassium, magnesium and calcium.

Consume Sufficient Good Salt.

In our society, it's said that reducing our sodium intake is important. A lot of people in our society are dealing with a high sodium / potassium ratio. This is due to the fact that we actually have higher insulin levels when we're on a higher carbohydrate diet. Insulin stimulates our kidneys so that sodium can be stored which can lead to a higher sodium or potassium ratio.

When we're on a low carbohydrate, ketogenic diet, we have lower levels of insulin and therefore our kidneys excrete much more sodium which can lead to lower sodium / potassium ratios and a greater dietary need for sodium.

Aim for an extra 3-5 grams of sodium from natural foods on a low-carb diet and using a pink salt such as Himalayan sea salt. 1 tsp of pink salt equals 2 g of sodium. Here are the ways to add sodium in addition and you'll find these are important ketogenic diet tips:.

- ❖ Drinking nutritious broth all day.
- ❖ Be generous with the consistency of sea salt or pink salt you use on the food.
- ❖ Add ¼ tsp of high-quality salt to 8-16 oz of water all day long.
- ❖ Adding to the dishes sea vegetables such as kelp, nori, and dulse.
- ❖ Consuming low carbon celery and cucumber with natural sodium.
- ❖ Use pumpkin seeds sprouted and salted or salted macadamia nuts as a snack.

Keep Stress Down.

Chronic stress will stop the ability to be in ketosis and stay in it. If you're going through a tough period of your life then it may not be the proper goal to maintain ketosis. This does not mean that you should start carb loading, but rather reset your target of simply staying on a low-carbon, anti-inflammatory diet.

Stress elevates stress hormones that work to elevate blood sugar, so you can fight or flee the chronic stressor. If it is for very short periods of time, this is fine, but when it is prolonged, it drives up your blood sugar then lowers ketones.

Create some techniques that can help you reduce your stress load and create more harmony and happiness in your life.

Don't Eat Too Much Of The Protein.

Many people who do a ketogenic diet eat too much protein. If you consume excessive protein then through a biochemical process called gluconeogenesis, your body may turn the amino acids into glucose.

You will eat tons of protein for some individuals and live in ketosis while others are unable to do so you have to learn and get to know your body.

If you see yourself coming out of ketosis then see how you respond to the protein in your meals. Some people need higher levels of protein while others may do just fine on lower levels of protein.

Key variables include your exercise level and exercise type (resistance vs aerobic) and your desire for muscle gain or weight loss. Someone who does rigorous muscle-gaining resistance training will need more protein than someone who's the same height and who's doing aerobic or resistance training to lose weight. Another person who weights the same but walks for exercise is going to need even less than the other two.

Ketogenic Diet Protein Consumption Tips.

- ❖ Measure your weight, and divide by 2.2 to calculate the protein grams per kg of body weight.
- ❖ Aim to get this on the lightest days of your workout. Bump it up to 1.6 gm/kg if you are doing more strength training or trying to gain muscle.
- ❖ Sedentary Body weight: 0.6-1.0 g / kg. If you're not exercising intensely, you may be struggling with 1 g / kg of protein to get into ketosis, so try dropping it back to 0.6-0.8 and seeing how you are doing.
- ❖ Active but not high intensity training: body weight 0.8-1.0 g / kg. If you walk regularly but do not do a high-intensity training (leaves you out of breath) or strength training then try 0.8 gram/kg and see what your ketone level looks like.

- ❖ Training at high intensity: 1.0-1.6 g / kg If you're weight training or doing workout style sprinting at least 3-4 days a week then you'll most likely need more than 1.0 g / kg. Try experimenting by bumpering it up to 1.2 g / kg and inch to 1.6 gram/kg and see how you feel and look like your ketone readings.
- ❖ With a minimum of 15 g & a maximum of 50 g per meal, it's ideal to get your protein in two (2)- three (3) different servings daily. The lower level is for an individual lightweight whilst the upper limit is for a very large male strength training.
- ❖ With a minimum of 15 gs and a maximum of 50 gs per meal, it's best to get your protein in 2-3 separate servings daily. The lower level is for an individual lightweight whilst the upper limit is for a very large male strength training.
- ❖ We should mostly aim for 20-35 grams per meal. Here's one example of how it would work:.

- ❖ Individual A: 150 lbs–require 68 grams of protein per day. Does not exercise except walks. This person should eat either 2 30-35 gram meals or 3 meals a day, with approximately 20-25 grams of protein per meal.
- ❖ Individual B: 150 lbs and loves performing 3-4x a week of resistance and aerobic exercise but they don't want to gain weight. This person should look for 68 grams on days of non-training, and 75-80 grams on days of training. So 25-30 grams of protein at mealtime.
- ❖ Individual C: 150lbs and performs 4-5x weekly high intensity resistance training and wants to gain muscle mass. On off days, they should consume around 80 grams of protein and on training days, 100 grams of protein. That would require 30-40 grams of protein per meal.

Stay Hydrated.

This is the most important ketogenic diet tips, but it is not always easy to follow. In our day to day lives we often get so distracted we fail to properly hydrate. Do super hydration of your body by consuming 32 oz of filtered water within the first waking hour and another 32-48 oz before midday.

Doing smoothies or keto coffee or tea, you can do a water fast or eat light in the morning. So the digestive system should tolerate well the hydration around these dishes. In general, it will benefit you tremendously to drink at least half of your body weight in ounces (Oz) of water and closer to your full body weight in ounces of water per day.

I weigh 160 lbs, and drink 140-180 ounces of water comfortably every day. Summertime sometimes more. Once you continue to hydrate your body more, you'll find that easier and easier, and you'll really be missing the extra hydration.

Using Mct Oil Any Time You Can.

Using a high-quality, medium chain triglyceride (MCT) oil may be the most important thing you can do to get into and sustain ketosis. That's because the use of a diet based on high MCT oil helps one to eat more protein / carbs and maintain ketosis.

A diet consisting of long-chain fatty acids relies on 80-90 per cent fat calories. Using tons of MCT oil decreases this to 60-70 per cent fat. This is because MCTs are quickly metabolized into ketone bodies and rapidly used in the body for energy.

Many people, including I, believe that coconut oil is identical to MCT oil for many years. It is not real. While MCT oil is made from coconut oil, it contains 100 percent pure medium chain triglycerides (caprylic acids and capric), while coconut oil contains approximately 35 percent long chain trigylceride (LCT) and 50 percent lauric acid, which is classically called a MCT but behaves more like an LCT. It means that coconut oil as pure MCT oil is only 15 per cent MCT and only 1/6th as ketogenic.

To keep your ketone levels up, you can cook with MCT oil, add it to protein shakes, green drinks, coffee / tea, and so on all day. Use our Keto Brain MCT oil which is the most ketogenic C8 caprylic acid on the market.

Keto Diet Recipes

Breakfast

Sheet Pan Eggs

Total time: 20 mins

Cook Time: 15 mins

Prep Time: 5 mins

Serves:6

Ingredients

- ❖ ¼ cup chopped chives
- ❖ Salt and pepper, to taste
- ❖ 12 large eggs
- ❖ ½ cup chopped mixed bell peppers
- ❖ Coconut oil, to grease the pan

Instructions

- ❖ Heat the oven up to 350 ° F. Grease a baking sheet measuring 12x17 inches with coconut oil.
- ❖ Whisk theeggs with salt and pepper in a large bowl until smooth.
- ❖ Add chopped chives and the mixed bell peppers.
- ❖ Pour the mixture in to the pan and bake for 12-15 minutes until set.
- ❖ Clean and let cool down slightly from the oven. Cut and serve squares.

Nutrition Info:

13 grams of protein, 2 grams of carbohydrates, 10 grams of fat

Paleo Breakfast Pizza

Prep Time: 10 minutes

Cook Time: 35 minutes

Total Time: 45 minutes

Servings 10 slices

Ingredients

For the crust:

- ❖ 2 tsp garlic powder
- ❖ 2 tsp Italian seasoning
- ❖ 6 large egg whites
- ❖ 1/2 cup coconut flour
- ❖ 1 cup coconut milk unsweetened
- ❖ 1 tsp onion powder
- ❖ 1/2 tsp baking soda

For the toppings:

- ❖ 1 cup baby spinach
- ❖ 1/2 tsp red pepper flakes
- ❖ 3 large eggs

- ❖ 1 tomato thinly sliced
- ❖ 1 tbsp extra virgin olive oil

Instructions

- ❖ Preheat an oven to 375 F.
- ❖ Prepare the large sheet of parchment paper for baking.
- ❖ Whisk the egg whites, seasonings, and coconut milk together in a large bowl. Then fold to combine in the coconut flour.
- ❖ Use a baking spatula to spread the dough over the prepared baking sheet to form a rectangle.
- ❖ Bake until the dough is firmly set for 15-18 minutes.
- ❖ Remove from the oven the crust and lower the oven to 350 degrees F.
- ❖ The extra virgin olive oil is spread over the crust using a baking brush or a spoon back. Spread the spinach, then the tomatoes, over the crush. Carefully smash the pizza with 3 eggs. Sprinkle with the flakes of red pepper.

Bake the egg whites in the oven for 12 minutes.

❖ Remove and devor from the oven!

Nutrition Info

Calories 121 kcal

Fat 8 g

Potassium 160 mg

Carbohydrates 5 g

Saturated Fat 5 g

Cholesterol 55 mg

Sodium 137 mg

Fiber 2 g

Sugar 1 g

Protein 5 g

Gluten Free Bacon and Egg Muffins

Prep/Cook Time: 30 mins,

Servings: 12

Ingredients

- ❖ 1/2 teaspoon(s) unrefined salt (I use THIS brand)
- ❖ many grinds of fresh black pepper
- ❖ coconut or ghee oil for oiling muffin liners
- ❖ 1/2 tsp garlic powder (like this)
- ❖ 10 eggs
- ❖ 6 strips of cooked bacon, then chopped into small pieces
- ❖ 1 teaspoon(s)
- ❖ ghee or coconut oil
- ❖ 2 cups spinach, chopped
- ❖ 2 tbsp fresh herbs (basil, cilantro, or parsley), finely chopped

Instructions

- ❖ Preheat 350'F oven. Line a silicone liner muffin pan or unbleached muffin liners. (I like to oil my silicone liners slightly.) Melt the fat of choice in a skillet over medium heat. Saute spinach until it starts to wilt for about a minute. Turn heat off. Add the pieces of chopped bacon and fresh herbs. Combine the mixture.
- ❖ Whisk 10 eggs, salt, pepper, and garlic powder in a large bowl. Place aside.
- ❖ Mix spinach / bacon spoon in your prepared cups of muffins. Pour over the mixture evenly with the whisked eggs.
- ❖ Bake for 20 minutes or until clean comes out the toothpick inserted into the center.

Creamy Cauliflower and Ground Beef Skillet

Prep/Cook Time: 40 mins

Serves: Serves 4

Ingredients

- ❖ 2 jalapeño peppers, sliced
- ❖ 1 tbsp fresh parsley, chopped
- ❖ 2 tsbp ghee (or make your own)
- ❖ ½ small onion, chopped
- ❖ 2 cloves garlic, chopped
- ❖ 1 small head cauliflower (454g, 1lb), grated
- ❖ ½ cup paleo mayo
- ❖ ½ cup water
- ❖ ¼ cup toasted sunflower seed butter
- ❖ 1 tbsp coconut aminos
- ❖ 4 jalapeño peppers, sliced
- ❖ 454g (1lb) lean ground beef
- ❖ 2 tbsp paleo mayo
- ❖ 1 tbsp apple cider vinegar
- ❖ 1 tsp fish sauce

- ❖ 1 tsp ground cumin
- ❖ 4 large eggs
- ❖ 1 tsp Himalayan salt
- ❖ ½ tsp freshly cracked black pepper
- ❖ ½ ripe avocado, diced

Instructions

- ❖ Melt ghee over medium-high heat in a heavy skillet (preferably cast iron). Add garlic, onion, and jalapeño pepper and cook until fragrant and soft, around 2-3 minutes, when the fat is nice and hot.
- ❖ Remove ground beef, salt and pepper and cook until the beef is red. Reduce heat to medium-low and throw in the rubbed cauliflower; stir well and cook for 2-3 minutes. (You can use your food processor's box grater to grate the coliflower.) In the meantime, add the mayo, water, sunflower butter, coconut amino, fish sauce and cumin to a large measuring cup then whisk until well mixed.

- ❖ Shink that over the ground beef and cauliflower mixture and stir until well absorbed. Continue cooking until all the liquid has been absorbed for about 3-5 minutes.
- ❖ Remove from heat, perfectly and uniformly distribute the meat mixture and create 4 shallow dimples. Sprinkle with salt, pepper, then
- ❖ jalapeño peppers in each of the dimples.
- ❖ Place your oven under the broiler for about 8-10 minutes or until the eggs are cooked to your taste.
- ❖ Alternatively, combine 2 mayo tablespoons with the vinegar of apple cider.
- ❖ Drizzle all over the frying pan as soon because it comes out of the oven, then garnish with fresh sliced parsley and diced avocado.
- ❖ Place the yolks and serve right away.

Coconut Flour Porridge

Prep Time: 2 minutes

Cook Time: 5 minutes

Total Time: 7 minutes

Servings 1

Ingredients

- ❖ 2 tablespoons golden flax meal
- ❖ 3/4 cup water
- ❖ 1 tablespoon Sukrin Gold or your favorite sweetener
- ❖ 1 large egg, beaten
- ❖ 2 teaspoons butter or ghee
- ❖ 2 tablespoons coconut flour
- ❖ pinch of salt
- ❖ 1 tablespoon heavy cream or coconut milk

Instructions

- ❖ Measure and stir the first four ingredients over medium heat into a small pot. Turn it down

- ❖ to medium-low when it begins to boil and whisk until it starts to thicken.
- ❖ Remove the porridge from the heat of the coconut flour and add the beaten egg, half at a time, whisking continuously. Return to heat and keep whisking before thickening of the porridge.
- ❖ Remove from heat and whisk before adding butter, cream and sweetener for about 30 seconds.
- ❖ Garnish with the toppings you need. (Net carbs of 4 grams)

Nutrition Info

Calories 345 Calories from Fat 257

Sugar 1.4g2%

Protein 13g26%

Fat 28.5g

Cholesterol 232mg

Carbohydrates 13g

Fiber 9g38%

Liver Sausage and Eggs

Total Time: 30 minutes

Cook Time: 30 minutes

Servings 4

Ingredients

- 1/2 pound(s) beef, ground
- 1/2 teaspoon(s) thyme, dried
- 1/4 pound(s) beef liver, ground
- 1 tablespoon(s) maple syrup
- 1 teaspoon(s) sage, dried
- 1/2 teaspoon(s) black pepper
- 2 tablespoon(s) olive oil
- 4 large egg(s)
- 1/2 teaspoon(s) rosemary, dried
- 1/2 teaspoon(s) sea salt
- 3/4 pound(s) pork, ground

Instructions

- In a large bowl, combine pork, beef, liver, maple syrup, seasonings and salt and pepper.

Mix with your hands until they are well combined and form into2-inch patties.

❖ In a pan heat half the olive oil and cook the patties until well browned and cooked. Cut the sausages, add the remaining oil to taste and fry the eggs. Serve with the willow.

Nutrition Info

calories 415, carbohydrate 5.6g, cholesterol 384mg, protein 52.6g, fat 19.3g, saturated fat 5.1g sodium 404mg, potassium 763mg, sugar 3.3g

Strawberry Avocado Keto Smoothie with Almond Milk

Prep Time: 2 minutes

Total Time: 2 minutes

Servings 1-cup servings

Ingredients

- ❖ 1 large Avocado
- ❖ 1/4 cup Erythritol
- ❖ 1 1/2 cup Unsweetened almond milk
- ❖ 1 lb Frozen strawberries

Instructions

Puree in a blender all ingredients until smooth. Adjust the sweetener as needed to taste.

Nutrition Info

Calories 106

Fat 7g

Total Carbs 12g

Net Carbs 7g

Protein 1g

Fiber 5g

Sugar 4g

Ground Beef, Eggs and Avocado Breakfast Bowl

Serves: Serves 1

Ingredients

- ❖ 6-8 medium mushrooms, sliced
- ❖ 150g grassfed ground beef
- ❖ 1 small onion, sliced
- ❖ 10-12 pitted black olives, sliced
- ❖ Salt and pepper to taste
- ❖ ½ tsp smoked paprika
- ❖ 2 eggs, lightly beaten
- ❖ 1 small avocado, diced

Instructions

- ❖ A little bit of coconut oil melts in a heavy skillet set over medium high heat. Add onions, mushrooms, salt and pepper when the oil is nice and hot and cook for 2-3 minutes until the veggies are fragrant and soft .

- ❖ Remove ground beef and smoked paprika and cook until the beef is not pink anymore. Take that away to a plate.
- ❖ Fill the skillet with eggs and scramble to your liking.
- ❖ Add the olives and the avocado then return the beef to the saucepan,
- ❖ Continue cooking for just about 45 seconds to a minute to warm up the avocados and olives.
- ❖ If needed, switch to a pretty cup, garnish with parsley, sit down and enjoy!

Guacamole Deviled Eggs

Total time: 10 mins

Prep Time: 10 mins

Serves:8

Ingredients

- ❖ 1 t garlic, minced
- ❖ 1 t shallot, minced
- ❖ 1 large avocado, very ripe
- ❖ 1 t lemon juice
- ❖ 6 hardboiled eggs, cooled and peeled
- ❖ 1/2 t paprika
- ❖ 3 T bacon bits
- ❖ pinch or two of salt
- ❖ pinch or two of pepper

Instructions

- ❖ Slice your eggs halfway through the length and spread over a baking sheet.
- ❖ Extract the yolks carefully from each egg and place a large bowl on them.

- ❖ In the bowl, add the avocado, garlic, bacon, shallot and lemon juice. Mash and stir until well combined.
- ❖ Taste the mixture to taste and season.
- ❖ Scoop the yolk and avocado mixture into the cavity of each slice of hardboiled egg using a small ice cream scoop, spoon or melon baller .
- ❖ Powder the paprika over each one, and enjoy!

Steak and Eggs

Prep Time: 10 minutes

Cook Time: 5 minutes

Servings: 1

Ingredients

- ❖ pepper
- ❖ 4 oz. sirloin
- ❖ 1/4 avocado
- ❖ 1 tbsp butter
- ❖ 3 eggs
- ❖ salt

Instructions

- ❖ Melt your butter in a saucepan then fry 2-3 eggs until the whites are set. Use salt and pepper to season.
- ❖ Cook your sirloin (or favorite steak cut) until desired doneness in another pan. Then season with salt and pepper in bite-sized strips.
- ❖ Slice up some of the avocado and serve!

Nutrition Info

510 Calories

36g of Fat

44g of Protein

3g of Net Carbs

Keto Breakfast Burger with Avocado Buns

Prep Time: 5 mins

Total time: 20 mins

Cook Time: 15 mins

Serves: 1 burger

Ingredients

- ❖ Sea salt, to taste
- ❖ Sesame seeds, for garnish
- ❖ 1 ripe avocado
- ❖ 1 egg
- ❖ 2 bacon rashers
- ❖ 1 tomato slice
- ❖ 1 lettuce leaf
- ❖ 1 T Paleo mayonnaise
- ❖ 1 red onion slice

Instructions

- ❖ Place the rashers of bacon on a cold frying pan. Switch on the stove and start to fry the bacon. Flip it with a fork as bacon beings curl. Continue to cook the bacon until it becomes crispy.
- ❖ Remove the bacon from the pan then use the bacon fat to cook the egg in the same bowl. Cook, but the yolk is still runny, until the white is set.
- ❖ Slice in half the size of the avocados. Remove the pit and scoop it out of your skin using a spoon.
- ❖ Fill the hole where Paleo mayonnaise used to be in the pit.
- ❖ Tomato, lettuce, onion, bacon, and fried egg layer.
- ❖ Season with salt from the sea.
- ❖ Top with the avocado's second half.
- ❖ Sprinkle with the seeds of sesame.

Nutrition Info

84 grams of protein, 121 grams of fat, 6 grams of carbohydrates,

Breakfast BLT Salad

Total Time: 15 mins

2 servings

Ingredients

- ❖ 3 cups shredded Lacinto kale, no stems
- ❖ 1 teaspoon red wine vinegar
- ❖ black pepper, to taste
- ❖ kosher salt
- ❖ 2 ounces sliced avocado
- ❖ 10 grape tomatoes, halved
- ❖ 2 large eggs
- ❖ 4 strips cooked center cut bacon, chopped
- ❖ 2 teaspoons extra virgin olive oil

Instructions

- ❖ Blend the kale, olive oil, vinegar and 1/4 teaspoon salt together in a bowl Massage about 3 minutes with your hands until the kale softens.

- ❖ I prefer soft boiled eggs to the perfect resemblance. How to make the perfect egg in the instant pot.
- ❖ Split the kale between two bowls, top with the following, tomatoes, avocado bacon, and egg.
- ❖ Complete with salt and pepper squeeze.

Nutrition Info

Calories: 292kcal, Fat: 18g, Carbohydrates: 18g, Saturated Fat: 4.5g, Protein: 17.5g

Snacks

Sugar Free Low Carb Keto Avocado Brownies

Prep Time: 10 minutes

Cook Time: 30 minutes

Total Time: 40 minutes

Servings 4

Ingredients

- ❖ 100 g (3.53 oz) lily's chocolate chips (1/2 cup (melted))
- ❖ 3 tabsp (3 tabsp) refined coconut oil (or butter, ghee, shortening, lard)
- ❖ 2 (2) eggs
- ❖ 250 g (8.82 ounces) avocado (1 cup mashed)
- ❖ 1/2 tsp (1/2 teasp) vanilla
- ❖ 4 tbsp (4 tabsp) cocoa powder

Dry Ingredients

- ❖ 90 g (3.17 ounces) blanched almond flour (3/4 cup)
- ❖ 1 tsp (1 tsp) stevia powder
- ❖ 1/4 tsp (1/4 teasp) baking soda
- ❖ 1/4 tsp (1/4 tsp) salt
- ❖ 60 ml (1/4 cups) erythritol
- ❖ 1 tsp (1 teasp) baking powder

Instructions

- ❖ The oven is preheated to 180C/350F.
- ❖ Mix the dry ingredients and whisk together in a separate bowl.
- ❖ Peel the lawyers. Weigh the avocados or weigh them. Place in a processor for food. Process until you are smooth.
- ❖ Adding each wet ingredient to the food processor, one at a time, and cycle until all the wet ingredients are added to the food processor for a few seconds.

- ❖ In the food processor, add the dry ingredients and mix until combined.
- ❖ Combine a piece of parchment paper to a 30x20 cm (12"x8"') baking dish and dump into the batter. Put the spoon in the preheated oven evenly. Bake for 30 minutes, or until half clean comes out a toothpick inserted in the centre. If you touch it with your fingers, the top should be soft.
- ❖ Remove from the oven and let it cool before slicing into 12 pieces.

Nutrition Info

Calories 155 Calories from Fat 126

Sugar 0.5g

Fat 14.05g

Saturated Fat 5.85g

Protein 4.02g

3 Ingredient Keto Peanut Butter Cookies

Servings: 4

Ingredients

- ❖ 1 cup peanut butter
- ❖ 1/2 cup keto sweetener of your choice
- ❖ 1 large egg

Instructions

- ❖ Pre-heat the oven to 350 ° C.
- ❖ Place all the ingredients in a bowl in a medium size bowl and mix everything until well mixed.
- ❖ Roll that dough into 1 inch balls using a scoop or your fingers.
- ❖ Place the dough balls on a parchment paper cookie sheet or silicone baking mat.
- ❖ Tip: Amazing are those silicone baking mats! Cookies are cooked evenly and every Time: the cookie crust is perfect! I highly recommend that you order this Silicone Baking Mat Set on

Amazon if you don't have any. It is well spent money!

- ❖ Press down twice in opposite directions on each ball with a fork to create a criss-cross pattern on each cookie
- ❖ You should bake these cookies for about 12 to 15 minutes or until golden brown.
- ❖ Allow them to cool before removing them from the tray for about 5 minutes.
- ❖ Save them in an airtight container if you have any left after the family gets a whiff of the wonderful scent that leads through the house and gets them standing over you in the kitchen just to wait to devour them!

Sugar Free Low Carb Keto Avocado Brownies

Prep Time: 10 minutes

Cook Time: 30 minutes

Total Time: 40 minutes

Servings 4 squares

Ingredients

- 100 g (3.53 oz) lily's chocolate chips (1/2 cup (melted))
- 3 tabsp (3 tabsp) refined coconut oil (or butter, ghee, shortening, lard)
- 250 g (8.82 ounces) avocado (1 cup mashed)
- 1/2 teasp (1/2 tsp) vanilla
- 4 tabsp (4 tabsp) cocoa powder
- 2 (2) eggs

Ingredients (Dry)

- 1 tsp (1 teasp) baking powder
- 1/4 tsp (1/4 teasp) salt

- ❖ 90 g (3.17 ounces) blanched almond flour (3/4 cup
- ❖ 1/4 teasp (1/4 tsp) baking soda
- ❖ 60 ml (1/4 cups) erythritol
- ❖ 1 tsp (1 teasp) stevia powder

Instructions

- ❖ Preheat to 180C/350F for the oven.
- ❖ Add dry ingredients together in a separate bowl and whisk together.
- ❖ Peel the lawyers. Weigh the avocados or weigh them. Put in a processor for meat. Process until you are smooth.
- ❖ Attach each wet ingredient to the food processor, one at a time, and process until all the wet ingredients are added to the food processor for a few seconds.
- ❖ In the food processor, add the dry ingredients and mix until combined.
- ❖ Put the piece of parchment paper over the baking dish measuring 30x20 cm (12"x8")

and pour in the batter. Place the spoon in the preheated oven evenly. Bake for 30 minutes or until half clean comes out a toothpick inserted in the centre. If you touch it with your fingers, the top should be soft.

❖ Remove from the oven and let it cool before slicing into 12 pieces.

Nutrition Info

Calories 155

Saturated Fat 5.85g37%

Potassium 140mg

Carbohydrates 9.78g

Fiber 6.98g

Sugar 0.5g1%

Protein 4.02g

Peanut Butter Power Granola

Prep Time: 10 mins

Cook Time: 30 mins

Total Time: 40 mins

Servings: 12 servings

Ingredients

- 1/4 cup butter
- 1/4 cup water
- 1 1/2 cups almonds
- 1 1/2 cups pecans
- 1 cup shredded coconut or almond flour
- 1/3 cup peanut butter
- 1/4 cup sunflower seeds
- 1/3 cup Swerve Sweetener
- 1/3 cup vanilla whey protein powder

Instructions

- Preheat oven to 300F and line with parchment paper a large rimmed baking sheet.

- ❖ Process almonds and pecans in a food processor until some larger pieces resemble coarse crumbs. Stir in shredded coconut, sunflower seeds, sweetener, and vanilla protein powder and move to a large bowl.
- ❖ Melt peanut butter & butter together in a safe bowl in a microwave.
- ❖ Pour the melted peanut butter over the mixture of the nut and stir well, slightly tossing. Remove the water. The mixture is going to clump together.
- ❖ On the prepared baking sheet, spread the mixture evenly and bake for 30 minutes. Remove and let it cool.

Nutrition Info

Calories 338 Calories from Fat 271

Fat 30.08g4

Carbohydrates 9.74g

Fiber 4.99g

Protein 9.36g

Lemon Strawberry Cheesecake Treats

Prep Time: 15 minutes

Total Time: 15 minutes

Servings 2

Ingredients

- ❖ 3 oz cream cheese, softened
- ❖ 3/4 cup heavy whipping cream
- ❖ 2 tspoons lemon extract
- ❖ zest of 1 lemon
- ❖ 2 large strawberries
- ❖ 1/3 cup Swerve sweetener

Instructions

- ❖ Add the cream cheese, sweetener and cream whipping in a mixing bowl. Beat up to smooth and creamy.
- ❖ Remove the juice of the lemon and blend well. If you want more lemon flavor add a bit of lemon zest as you're not going to need it all.

- ❖ Take 1 of the strawberries and cut into small pieces. Slice into small heart-shaped pieces with the other strawberry.
- ❖ Fill half way each jar with half the mixture of cream cheese.
- ❖ To make a nice layer, add the chopped strawberry to both bottles.
- ❖ Fill with the rest of the cream cheese mixture the strawberries.
- ❖ Use the strawberry slices to create a flow pattern at the top.
- ❖ In the middle of each flower, sprinkle the lemon zest. You don't need to use all the zest, which just looks nice.
- ❖ Cool until ready to eat.

Note: Any sweetener you like can be used. Just make sure you use 1/3 cup sugar in the same quantity.

Nutrition Info

474 cals, 0.4g fiber, 5.7g carbs, 48.2g fat, 4.5g protein

Classic Chocolate Cake Donuts

Prep Time: 15 mins

Cook Time: 18 mins

Total Time: 33 mins

Servings: 8

Ingredients

Donuts

- ❖ 1/3 cup Swerve Sweetener
- ❖ 3 tablesp cocoa powder
- ❖ 1/4 cup butter melted
- ❖ 1/2 teasp vanilla extract
- ❖ 1 tsp baking powder
- ❖ 1/4 teasp salt
- ❖ 4 large eggs
- ❖ 1/3 cup coconut flour
- ❖ 6 tablesp brewed coffee or water coffee intensifies the chocolate flavour

Glaze:

- 1 tbsp heavy cream
- 1/4 tsp vanilla extract
- 1/4 cup powdered Swerve Sweetener
- 1 tbsp cocoa powder
- 1 1/2 to 2 tbsp water

Instructions

Donuts:

- Pre-heat oven to 325F then grease a donut pan very well.
- Whisk the coconut flour, sweetener, cocoa powder, baking powder, and salt together in a medium bowl. Add the potatoes, butter melted, and vanilla extract, then stir in the cold coffee or water until well combined.
- Divide the batter between the donut pan wells. You may need to work in loads if you have a six-well donut pan.

- ❖ Bake until the donuts are set and firm to the touch for 16 to 20 mins. Remove & let it cool for 10 min in the pan, then turn over a wire rack to cool completely.
- ❖ Glaze: Whisk together the powdered sweetener and cocoa powder in a medium shallow bowl. Add the heavy vanilla and cream and whisk together.
- ❖ Add enough water, without being too watery, until the glaze thins out and has a "dippable" texture.
- ❖ Dip into the glaze the top of each donut and set for about 30 minutes.

Nutrition Info

Calories 123 Calories from Fat 83

Fiber 2.67g

Fat 9.2g

Carbohydrates 4.68g

Protein 4.43g

Pistachio toffee cups

Prep Time: 10 minutes

Cook Time: 10 minutes

Total Time: 20 minutes

Yield: 15 candies

Ingredients

- ❖ Salt to taste
- ❖ 3 Tabsp unsalted butter
- ❖ ½ ounce raw pistachios, chopped
- ❖ 5 ounces low carb chocolate
- ❖ 3 Tabsp + 2 tsp sweetener of your choice
- ❖ 1/2 teasp vanilla extract

Instructions

- ❖ You have to melt half of the chocolate very slowly in a double boiler or microwave at half-power in a small bowl at 10 second intervals, stirring frequently and testing periodically to ensure that it does not scorch. This could take

30 seconds, so be careful to watch it. Save for later the other half of the chocolate.

❖ Brush that melted chocolate on the bottom and sides in a thin layer using a pastry brush or a spoon in a cupcake tray filled with cupcake liners (or a silicone candy mold).

❖ Freeze the mold until the chocolate sets for about ten minutes.

❖ Add the butter and sweetener in another small bowl. Melt at low power in the microwave (I used level 3) at intervals of 10 seconds, stirring frequently. It will start bubbling (like brown butter) and smell nutty. Remove from the microwave when it starts to get darker and tan in color. The bowl is going to be very warm, so be careful. Immediately add the vanilla and chopped pistachios and stir in two more teaspoons of sweetener.

❖ Working fast (hardening quickly), spooning half a teaspoon or more of the toffee mixture into each mold of chocolate.

- ❖ Once filled, microwave as with the first batch the rest of the chocolate, making sure not to scorch it. Cover and smooth each candy with a little chocolate.
- ❖ If you like, sprinkle with salt. For at least an hour, freeze or chill the candies and place in the refrigerator. Live!

Notes.

You can make use of any type of nut, any type of extract of flavor (almond would be nice!), and any type of chocolate. I used Lily's milk chocolate as a low carb option, but white chocolate will work any way. Stevia or erythritol works well for a toffee-free sugar option.

Keto Coconut Mocha Doughnuts

Prep Time: 10 minutes

Cook Time: 20 minutes

Total Time: 30 minutes

Servings: 6 Doughnuts

Ingredients

- 1/2 teasp baking powder
- 1/2 teasp baking soda
- 4 eggs
- 1/4 cup coconut oil
- 3 Tabsp unsweetened cocoa powder
- 1 Tbsp liquid stevia
- 1/2 teasp instant coffee granules
- 1/3 cup coconut flour
- 1/3 cup not sweet almond milk (or coconut milk)

Instructions

- The oven should be preheated to 350.

- ❖ Inside a mixing bowl, combine all ingredients and mix well.
- ❖ Mix and bake for 20 minutes in a doughnut pan.
- ❖ Place on a rack for cooling and let it cool.
- ❖ Serve and make the most of it! A great mug of coffee or non-daily milk is going well!

Nutrition Info

Calories: 707 Carbohydrates: 17g Total Fat: 66g, Protein: 19g

Keto Cinnamon Roll Biscotti

Prep Time: 20 mins

Cook Time: 1 hr

Total Time: 1 hr 20 mins

Servings: 15 biscotti

Ingredients

Filling/Topping:

- 1 tsp ground cinnamon
- 2 tbsp Swerve Sweetener

Biscotti:

- 1 tsp vanilla extract
- 1 large egg
- 2 cups almond flour Honeyville
- 1/3 cup Swerve Sweetener
- 1/4 tsp salt
- 1/4 cup melted butter plus 1 tbsp for brushing biscotti
- 1 tsp baking powder

- ❖ 1/2 tsp xanthan gum

Glaze:

- ❖ 1/2 tsp vanilla
- ❖ 1/4 cup powdered Swerve Sweetener
- ❖ 2 tbsp heavy cream

Instructions

For filling

- ❖ Combine sweetener and cinnamon in a little bowl for filling. Set aside.
- ❖ Preheat the oven to 325F and line a parchment paper baking sheet.
- ❖ Whisk the almond flour, sweetener, baking powder, xanthan gum, and salt together in a large bowl. Add the butter, egg and vanilla extract 1/4 cup until the dough is combined.
- ❖ Turn the dough onto the baking sheet prepared and divide in half. Shape every half into a 10-by-4-inch rectangle. Make sure the size and shape of both halves are similar.

- ❖ Sprinkle with about 2/3 of the filling of cinnamon one half. Seal the edges & smooth the surface with the other half of the flour.
- ❖ Bake for 25 minutes or until the touch is slightly browned and firm. Remove the remaining melted butter from the oven and comb, then dust with the remaining mixture of cinnamon. Let it cool for 30 minutes and lower the oven to 250F.
- ❖ Cut the log into about 15 slices using a sharp knife (a straight up and down motion works better than looking back and forth).
- ❖ Place slices on the cut-side down baking sheet and bake for 15 minutes, then turn over and bake for another 15 minutes. Switch off the oven then let it sit until it's cool inside.
- ❖ For the glaze, whisk the cream and vanilla extract powdered sweetener until smooth. Drizzle over refrigerated biscotti.

Nutrition Info

133 Calories; 12g Fat (79.0% calories from fat); 4g Protein; 2g Dietary Fiber; 27mg Cholesterol; 4g Carbohydrate; 113mg Sodium.

Jenni Treesong

Avocado Popsicle with Coconut & Lime

Prep Time: 5 minutes

Cook Time: 3 minutes

Total Time: 8 minutes

Servings: 6 Servings

Ingredients

- ¼ cup erythritol Granular Swerve sweeter
- 2 tablespoons lime juice
- 2 avocados pitted
- 1.5 cups coconut milk

Instructions

- Place in a blender all ingredients; secure lid and pulse to break down ingredients.
- Scrape the blender's internal sides to add splattered ingredients and remove the cap.
- Blend without lumps until the mixture is smooth, creamy.

- ❖ Distribute the mixture evenly into six molds of the popsicle. The mixed ingredients are thick; it may be easier to spoon the mixture into the molds than to pour.
- ❖ To remove air bubbles & settle the mixture, tap the filled molds on the counter top.
- ❖ In the center of the molds, place popsicle sticks or handles in the mixture.
- ❖ For several hours, freeze the molds until the mixture has completely solidified.
- ❖ Push the mold briefly under water when you're ready to eat to help release the popsicle. Gently pull the handle out of the popsicle and enjoy!

Notes: For the recipe, choose a low fat or lite coconut milk to minimize dietary fat and calories.

Nutrition Info

Calories: 219kcal, Carbohydrates: 8g, Protein: 2g Sodium: 12mg, Fat: 21g, Saturated Fat: 12g, Potassium: 449mg

Classic Blueberry Scones

Prep Time: 15 mins

Cook Time: 25 mins

Total Time: 40 mins

Servings: 12

Ingredients

- 3/4 cup fresh blueberries
- 1/3 cup Swerve Sweetener
- 1/4 cup coconut flour
- 1 tbsp baking powder
- 1/4 tsp salt
- 2 large eggs
- 1/4 cup heavy whipping cream
- 2 cups almond flour
- 1/2 tsp vanilla extract

Instructions

- Pre-heat the oven to 325F and line a large parchment or silicone liner baking sheet.

- ❖ Whisk the almond flour, sweetener, coconut flour, baking powder, and salt together in a large bowl.
- ❖ Remove the eggs, whipping the cream and vanilla, and mix until the dough starts to come together. Add the blueberries to the dough and work carefully.
- ❖ Assemble the dough and transfer onto the prepared baking sheet. Pat about 10 by 8 inches in a rough rectangle.
- ❖ To cut into 6 squares, use a sharp, large knife. Then diagonally cut each of these squares into two triangles. Lift the scones gently and spread them around the pan.
- ❖ Bake for 20minutes to 25 minutes, until brown and firm to the touch. Remove, let it cool.

Nutrition Info

Calories 153 Calories from Fat 109

Fat 12.15g

Carbohydrates 7.21g

Fiber 3.06g

Protein 5.55g

Salad And Side Dish

Peanut Butter & Jam Cups

Prep Time: 5 mins

Cook Time: 10 mins

Chill Time: 45 mins

Total Time: 15 mins

Servings: 12

Ingredients

- ❖ 3/4 cup raspberries
- ❖ 6 to 8 tablesp powdered Swerve Sweetener divided
- ❖ 1/4 cup water
- ❖ 1 teasp grassfed gelatin
- ❖ 3/4 cup creamy peanut butter
- ❖ 3/4 cup coconut oil

Instructions

- Line a 12 silicone or parchment paper liner on muffin pan.
- Combine the raspberries with water in a medium saucepan over medium heat. Take to boil, lower the heat and simmer for 5 minutes. With a fork, mash the berries.
- Remove the powdered sweetener from 2 to 4 tbsp, depending on how sweet you like it. Whisk the grassfed gelatin and let the peanut butter mixture cool while it is being prepared.
- Add the peanut butter & coconut oil in a microwave safe bowl. Cook 30 to 60 seconds on high, until melted. Depending on how hot you like it, whisk the powdered sweetener in 2 to 4 tbsp (I only use 2 tbsp).
- Divide half of the mixture of peanut butter among the twelve cups and set about 15 minutes in the freezer to firm up. Divide between the cups the raspberry mixture and

top with the remaining mixture of peanut butter.

❖ Refrigerate to firm. Keep it refrigerated.

Nutrition Info

Calories 223 Calories from Fat 196

Fat 21.77g

Carbohydrates 4.52g

Fiber 1.31g

Protein 3.84g

Jenni Treesong

Homemade Caramel Frappuccino

Prep Time: 5 mins

Total Time: 5 mins

Servings: 1 very large

Ingredients

- 1 1/2 cups crushed ice
- 1/4 tsp caramel flavour
- 1/2 cup unsweetened almond milk
- 1/4 cup heavy whipping cream
- 1 tsp instant espresso powder
- Lightly sweetened whipped cream for topping
- 10 drops liquid stevia extract

Instructions

- Combine whipping cream, coffee, ice, almond milk, stevia extract, and caramel flavor in a high-powered blender like a Blendtec.
- Mix until it is smooth.
- Top with a whipped cream.

Nutrition Info

Calories 273 Calories from Fat 247

Total fat: 27.40g

Sodium: 117mg

Carbohydrate: 2.99g

Total dietary fiber: 0.50g

Calories from fat: 246

Cholesterol: 101mg

Protein: 2.15g

Keto Broccoli Salad with Bacon

Prep Time: 5 minutes

Cook Time: 2 minutes

Total Time: 7 minutes

Servings 6

Ingredients

- ❖ 2 Tbspoons apple cider vinegar
- ❖ 1/4 cup onion , chopped (optional)
- ❖ 3 stevia packets
- ❖ 1/4 cup roasted sunflower seeds (optional)
- ❖ 1/2 cup cheddar cheese , grated
- ❖ 1 bunch fresh broccoli , cut in small pieces
- ❖ 3/4 cup mayonnaise
- ❖ 6 slices no sugar bacon , cooked crisp and chopped

structions

- ❖ For a minute or two minutes, steam the broccoli lightly. Drain and cool.
- ❖ Mix mayonnaise, vinegar and stevia in a big bowl with a whisk.
- ❖ Toss in the dressing the broccoli and cheddar cheese.

Notes.

- ❖ Simply omit the cheese to make the salad dairy-free.
- ❖ The salad can be changed by adding dried cranberries that are free of sugar or nuts.

Nutrition Info

Calories: 390kcal, Saturated Fat: 8g, Fat: 36g, Carbohydrates: 9g, Protein: 9g, Cholesterol: 36mg, Sodium: 416mg

Keto Carrot Cake

Prep Time: 10 minutes

Cook Time: 2 minutes

Total Time: 12 minutes

Servings 2 Servings

Ingredients

For the cake

- ❖ 1/4 teasp ground cloves (optional)
- ❖ 1 tabsp melted butter
- ❖ 2 tbsp almond flour
- ❖ 1 tabsp psyllium husk
- ❖ 1/2 teasp baking powder
- ❖ 1 tabsp erythritol
- ❖ 1/2 teasp vanilla extract
- ❖ 1/2 small carrot finely grated
- ❖ pinch of salt
- ❖ 1 teasp cinnamon
- ❖ 1 large egg lightly beaten

- ❖ 1/4 teasp ground ginger

For the frosting

- ❖ 1/2 tsp vanilla extract
- ❖ 1/4 cp cream cheese at room temperature
- ❖ 1 tbsp whipping cream
- ❖ 1/2 tabsp erythritol

Instructions

- ❖ Combine all the ingredients of your cake in a mug and thoroughly mix until all is well incorporated. It may also be done in a blender or food processor. Microwave for 90 seconds at high heat. Remove your cake from the mug and let it cool down completely. Slice your cake to make two layers and put them in a cool place.
- ❖ Add cream cheese, erythritol and extract of vanilla in a bowl. Use an electric hand blender to whip all the ingredients to produce a smooth creamy blend. Attach the whipping

cream and play for another 5 minutes. Set aside.
- ❖ Take a cake layer and scoop a heaped tbsp of your frosting cream cheese on top of it. Place the top layer gently on it and scoop up another heaped tbsp of frosting cream cheese. Spread the leftover frosting in any direction you want by using the back for the spoon.
- ❖ Serve immediately or chill before serving. The warmer the cake gets, the heavier the icing is going to be, and vice versa.

Nutrition Info

Calories: 229kcal, Protein: 6g, Fat: 17.3g, Carbohydrates: 20g, Fiber: 15.9g

Keto Lemon Bars

Prep Time: 15 minutes

Cook Time: 45

Total Time: 1 hour

8 servings

Ingredients

- ❖ 1 cup powdered erythritol, divided
- ❖ 3 medium lemons
- ❖ 3 large eggs
- ❖ 1/2 cup butter, melted
- ❖ 1 3/4 cups almond flour, divided

Instructions

- ❖ Mix together butter, 1 cup of almond flour, 1/4 cup of erythritol and a pinch of salt. Push uniformly into a paper-lined baking dish with a parchment of 8 segments8". Bake at 350 ° F for 20 minutes. Then let 10 minutes cool down.

- Add the eggs, 3/4 cup erythritol, 3/4 almond flour & pinch of salt to a pan, zest one of the lemons, then juice all 3 lemons. Combine in order to fill.
- Pour over the filling and bake for 25 minutes.
- Serve with slices of lemon and an erythritol sprinkle.

Notes

If you're used to adding vanilla extract to crust, feel free to mix 1/2 tsp into the crust.

Nutrition Info

Serving Size: 1 bar

Calories: 272

Carbohydrates: 4g net

Protein: 8g

Fat: 26g

iflower Casserole with

…utes

Cook Time: 45 minutes

Total Time: 55 minutes

Servings: 6 Servings

Ingredients

- ❖ 1/2 teaspoon salt
- ❖ 1/2 teaspoon ground pepper
- ❖ 6 cups cauliflower florets
- ❖ 4 teaspoons olive oil
- ❖ 1 teaspoon dried oregano
- ❖ 2 ounces goat cheese chevre, crumbled

The Sauce:

- ❖ 28 ounce can of crushed tomatoes
- ❖ 2 bay leaves
- ❖ 1/4 teaspoon salt
- ❖ 1 teaspoon olive oil

- ❖ 1/4 cup minced flat-leaf parsley
- ❖ 3 garlic cloves minced

Instructions

- ❖ Preheat the oven to 425 F.
- ❖ Combine the cauliflower seeds, olive oil, oregano, salt and pepper on a baking sheet. Toss to dress up.
- ❖ When pierced with a fork, roast until the cauliflower is barely tender, turning occasionally, about 25 minutes.
- ❖ Coat lightly with cooking spray a 7-by 11-inch baking dish. In the baking dish, put the roasted cauliflower and top with the marinara sauce and crumbled goat cheese.
- ❖ Bake for about 20 minutes until the cauliflower is soft and the goat cheese is melted. Honor. Serve.
- ❖ The sauce: warm the olive oil over medium heat in a large non-stick skillet. Add the garlic and bake, stirring constantly for 30 seconds.

❖ Remove the crushed tomatoes and leaves from the bay. Take to the boil and cook for 15 minutes. Cut the leaves of the bay and dump them. Stir in the parsley and butter.

Nutrition Info

Calories: 127.7kcal, ,

Carbohydrates: 16g, Protein: 5.7g , Cholesterol: 3.3mg, Fat: 6.4g, Saturated Fat: 1.9g Sodium: 540.2mg, Fiber: 5.2g, Sugar: 7.8g

Jenni Treesong

Mexican Cauliflower "Rice"

Prep Time: 10 min

Cook Time: 5 min

Total Time: 15 min

Ingredients

- ❖ Salt & Pepper, to taste
- ❖ 1 Head Small/Medium Cauliflower, I used orange cauliflower, but white works just as well!
- ❖ 1 Tablespoon Extra-Light Olive Oil
- ❖ 1 Small Onion, finely chopped
- ❖ 2 Cloves Garlic, finely minced
- ❖ 2 Tablespoons Tomato Paste (make sure there's no added sugar
- ❖ 1 Tablespoon Ghee*
- ❖ ½ Cup Chicken Broth, or vegetable broth
- ❖ Fresh Cilantro Leaves, for garnish

Instructions

- ❖ Use a box grater or the grating device to grate the cauliflower on a food processor. Put it aside.
- ❖ Heat oil and ghee over high heat in a large skillet and throw in the garlic and onion; sauté for 2 minutes or until soft and fragrant. Add the tomato paste and add salt and pepper to the mixture.
- ❖ Add the chicken broth and the cauliflower and blend well. Cover for 3 minutes and cook.
- ❖ Remove from heat the cauliflower rice and garnish with coriander. Serve with any of Mexico's favorite dishes!

Cheddar Bacon Cauliflower Potato Salad

Prep Time: 10 minutes

Cook Time: 5 minutes

Total Time: 15 minutes

Servings: 6

Ingredients

- 1/2 teaspoon salt
- 1/2 teaspoon pepper
- 6 slices fried bacon, diced
- 2 hard boiled eggs, peeled and diced
- 1 tablespoon dill
- 1 large head cauliflower
- ½ cup grated cheddar
- ⅓ cup mayonnaise
- 1/4 cup chopped red onion
- 1 teaspoon mustard

Instructions

- ❖ Cut the coliflower into pieces of bite size and place it in a basket of steamers.
- ❖ Steam until tender-crisp for 3-5 minutes.
- ❖ Put cauliflower in the large mixing bowl and chill for 2 hours in the refrigerator.
- ❖ In the cauliflower bowl, add the remaining ingredients and stir well to combine.
- ❖ Serve right away.

Nutrition Info

Calories: 210 Sodium: 463mg, Saturated Fat: 5g Trans Fat: 0g Unsaturated Fat: 11g Total Fat: 17gCholesterol: 82mg Carbohydrates: 8g Fiber: 3g Sugar: 4g Protein: 9g

Low Carb Macaroni Salad

Prep Time: 10 minutes

Cook Time: 5 minutes

Total Time: 15 minutes

Servings 1

Ingredients

- 1 cup raw cauliflower broken into very small pieces
- 1 tspoon of grated carrot
- 3 tspoons salad olives
- 1 to 2 tbspoons sugar free Mayonnaise
- 1/2 teaspoon cider vinegar optional
- Pinch of salt
- Stevia or other sweetener to taste
- 1 tspoon Dijon mustard
- 2 tbpoons of thinly sliced celery
- 1 tablespoon of bell pepper
- Pinch of pepper
- 2 tspoons of chopped onion

Instructions

- ❖ Steam the cauliflower until very tender, but not to mushy.
- ❖ Mix mayonnaise, mustard, vinegar, salt, pepper and sweetener together and mix well.
- ❖ Seasoning taste and adjust.
- ❖ In a bowl, place cauliflower, celery, carrot, onion, pepper and olives.
- ❖ Pour over the mayonnaise mixture and gently combine.
- ❖ Chill over overnight or longer.
- ❖ When necessary, add a little more dressing before serving.

Nutrition Info

Calories: 80kcal, Protein: 2g, Fat: 4g, Carbohydrates: 8g, Saturated Fat: 0g

Jenni Treesong

Cheesy Cauliflower alla Vodka Casserole

8 servings

Ingredients

- ❖ 6 slices Provolone cheese
- ❖ 1/4 cup fresh basil, chopped
- ❖ 8 cups cooked cauliflower florets, well drained
- ❖ 2 cups vodka sauce
- ❖ 2 Tbsp heavy whipping cream
- ❖ 1/3 cup grated Parmesan cheese
- ❖ 1/2 tsp kosher salt
- ❖ 1/4 tsp ground black pepper
- ❖ 2 Tbsp melted butter

Instructions

- ❖ Combine in a large bowl the cauliflower, vodka sauce, heavy cream whipping, butter, Parmesan cheese, kosher salt, and black pepper, and toss well.

- ❖ Transfer to (or equivalent) a 9x 13 baking dish and top with Provolone (or mozzarella) cheese slices.
- ❖ Bake for 30 –40 minutes in a preheated 375 degree (F) oven or until the casserole bubbles and the cheese is melted.
- ❖ Switch from the oven for about 10 minutes and let it rest.
- ❖ Top and serve with chopped fresh basil.

Nutrition info

214 calories, 12g protein, 14g fat, 6g net carbs,

Lunch And Dinr

Loaded Chicken Salad

Prep Time: 10 minutes

Cook Time: 8 minutes

Total Time: 18 minutes

Ingredients

- ❖ 1 tsp extra virgin olive oil
- ❖ 1/4 tsp Himalayan salt
- ❖ 1/2 red onion
- ❖ 5 asparagus
- ❖ 1/4 tsp black pepper
- ❖ 1 har artichoke hearts
- ❖ 1 avocado
- ❖ 100 g mozzarella balls
- ❖ 1 large tomato (any colour)
- ❖ 1 boneless chicken breast (with or without skin about 300g)
- ❖ 20 leaves basil

- ❖ 4 cups baby spinach (200g used)

Dressing

- ❖ 1 tsp dijon mustard
- ❖ 1 clove garlic
- ❖ pinch black pepper
- ❖ pinch Himalayan salt
- ❖ 2 tbsp extra virgin olive oil
- ❖ 1 1/2 tbsp balsamic vinegar

Instructions

- ❖ Peel the avocado and dice it. Slice the onion in the red. Tomato dice. Bring together the basil leaves, roll them up and cut them. Cut off the asparagus stems and cut in half. Slim the garlic.
- ❖ Slice the breast of the chicken in half. Sprinkle on each hand the 1/4 tsp of pepper and salt . Inside a cast iron skillet, heat 1 tbsp of olive oil and put the chicken breasts in. Fry on each side, about 3 minutes per side, until golden

brown and cooked through. Place the asparagus next to the breasts of the chicken and cook until soft and grilled for a few minutes. Bring the slice and the chicken out.

- ❖ Combine chopped garlic, olive oil, balsamic vinegar, dijon, and salt & peper in a small bowl.
- ❖ In a large bowl or pan, add the baby spinach. Cover with chicken grilled, avocado, mozzarella, tomatoes, artichoke, red onions, asparagus and leaves of basil. Pour over and enjoy the styling!

Note

If you don't care for extra carbs or want a sweeter dressing, you can add 1 tbsp of honey to the salad dressing.

Nutrition Info

Calories 430 Calories from Fat 264

Total Carbohydrates 12.86g 4%

Dietary Fiber 6.12g 24%

Total Fat 29.36g 45%

Saturated Fat 6.57g 33%

Sugars 3.16g

Protein 31.73g 63%

Crack Slaw Egg Roll in a Bowl

Cook Time: 15 minutes

Total Time: 15 minutes

Servings servings (1 cup each)

Ingredients

- ❖ 1 tbsp Sea salt
- ❖ 4 cloves Garlic (minced)
- ❖ 1 tbp Avocado oil
- ❖ 3 tbs Fresh ginger (minced or grated; or use 3/4 tsp ground ginger)
- ❖ 1/4 tbsp Black pepper (or more if you want it spicy)
- ❖ 1 lb Ground beef
- ❖ 2 tbsp Toasted sesame oil
- ❖ 1/4 cup Green onions
- ❖ 1 lb Shredded coleslaw mix (~4 cups)
- ❖ 1/4 cup Coconut aminos

Instructions

- ❖ Heat the avocado oil Over a medium to high heat in a large saute pan. Add ginger and garlic. Saute until fragrant, for about a minute.
- ❖ Add the beef to the ground. Season with black pepper and sea salt. Cook for about 7-10 minutes until browned.
- ❖ Reduce to medium heat. Apply the aminos of coleslaw and coconut. Remove to coat. Cook until cabbage is tender for about 5 minutes.
- ❖ Take off the heat. Attach the toasted oil of sesame and green onions.

Nutrition Info

Protein 15g

Total Carbs 8g

Calories 231

Fat 15g

Net Carbs 4g

Fiber 4g

Sesame Salmon w. Baby Bok Choy & Mushrooms

Serving: 4

Ingredients

Main Dish

- ❖ 2 each portobello mushroom caps (or 8 ounces. baby bella mushrooms)
- ❖ 4 each baby bok choy
- ❖ 4 each 4-6 ounces. salmon fillet
- ❖ 1 tbp toasted sesame seeds
- ❖ 1 ea green onion

Marinade

- ❖ 1/2 tbsp black pepper
- ❖ 1 tbs Coconut Aminos
- ❖ 1/2 lemon juice
- ❖ 1 tbs olive oil
- ❖ 1 tsp sesame oil
- ❖ 1/2 inch Ginger grated 1 tsp.
- ❖ 1/2 tbsp Salt

Instructions

- ❖ Whisk all of the marinade ingredients together Drizzle half of the salmon marinade and turn to coat. Cover and refrigerate the salmon during one hour of marinating.
- ❖ Heat the oven up to 400.
- ❖ Prepare vegetables: cut in half the rough ends of the bok choy. Cut the mushrooms into pieces of 1/2 inch.
- ❖ Drizzle over the vegetables with the remaining marinade and lay on a lined baking sheet.
- ❖ Place the salmon on a sheet of lined baking, skin side down. Bake until the salmon is cooked through for about 20 minutes.
- ❖ Top with green sliced onions and seeds of sesame.

Low Carb Keto Chili

Prep Time: 5 minutes

Cook Time: 30 minutes

Total Time: 35 minutes

Servings: 6

Ingredients

- 1 tsp ground chipotle chili powder
- 1 tbsp chili powder
- 1/2 tbsp avocado oil
- 2 ribs celery, chopped
- 2 lbs. 85/15 ground beef
- 1 tsp salt
- 1 tsp black pepper
- 1 15 oz. can no-salt-added tomato sauce
- 1 16.2 oz. container Kettle & Fire Beef Bone Broth
- 2 tsp garlic powder
- 1 tbsp cumin

Instructions

- ❖ Over medium
- ❖ in a large pot, heat. Heat avocado oil . Add the chopped celery and cook for about 3-4 minutes until softened. To separate the bowl, transfer the celery and set aside.
- ❖ Add beef and spices and brown beef in the same pot until all is cooked.
- ❖ Reduce to medium-low heat, stirring occasionally, add tomato sauce and beef bone broth to cooked beef, and cook covered for 10 minutes.
- ❖ Return the celery to the pot and swirl until well integrated.
- ❖ Garnish, serve, and have fun!

Nutrition Info

Serving Size: 1 cup

Calories: 359

Protein: 34.4g

Fat: 22.8g

Carbohydrates: 6.7g (Net: 5.2g)

Lemon Balsamic Chicken

Prep Time: 5 minutes

Cook Time: 30 minutes

Total Time: 35 minutes

Servings: 6

Ingredients

- 1 cup shredded purple cabbage
- 2 tbsp. minced lemon rind
- 2 bay leaves
- 8 chicken thighs (about 2 lbs) skinless boneless
- 3 tbsp. pastured butter
- 1 cup sliced onion
- 2 tsp pink Himalayan salt
- 1 tsp dried Italian herb blend
- 5 tbsp. olive oil
- 1 tsp coarse black pepper
- 1.5 tbsp. balsamic vinegar

Instructions

- ❖ In sauté mode, steam your electrical pressure cooker. put 2 cbsp. Cream. Butter.
- ❖ Peel and cut the onion as it melts. Go ahead and prepare your cabbage and lemon rind as well!
- ❖ Apply to the stress the onion, cabbage and lemon. Sauce, sometimes stirring until tender.
- ❖ Apply wings, seasonings and leaves of the bay to the chicken. Remove well and cook for 2-3 minutes, browning the chicken.
- ❖ Verse the vinegar. Cancel the role of a sauté. Close the lid, choose the cook pressure. Set it for 20 minutes in the poultry or high.
- ❖ Let the pressure release naturally once it's finished. Open the lid, stir to shred the chicken. Pour in butter's last teaspoon.
- ❖ Sprinkle this wonderful sauce chicken with olive oil or avocado oil all over your zoodles! Love! Enjoy!

Nutrition Info

Calories: 325

Fat: 17.8

Carbohydrates: 6.9

Fiber: 4

Protein: 29

Salmon Gremolata with Roasted Vegetables

Prep Time: 10 minutes

Cook Time: 20 minutes

Total Time: 30 minutes

Servings: 4

Ingredients

- 4 salmon fillets

GREMOLATA

- 1 lemon, zested
- 1 cup almond flour
- 1 tbsp olive oil
- 2 cloves garlic
- 1/4 cup parsley leaves
- salt
- pepper

ROASTED VEGETABLES (optional)

- 1 tbsp olive oil

- ❖ Salt
- ❖ 1 bunch asparagus
- ❖ 1 cup cherry tomatoes
- ❖ pepper

Instructions

- ❖ Heat the oven to 350F for a fan oven, 380F for a non-fan oven.
- ❖ Blitz the garlic, parsley and almond meal in a blender or food processor and stir in the lemon zest.
- ❖ Place salmon filets on a greased or parchment lined sheet pan.
- ❖ Season the salmon filets with salt and pepper, brush or sprinkle with a little oil, then carefully press the Gremolata crumb mixture to the top.
- ❖ If you use the optional vegetables to roast alongside the salmon, simply pour them in a little oil, place them around the salmon in the pan and season with salt and pepper.

❖ Bake for about 15 minutes-20 minutes until the fish is cooked through and the tops are golden.

Nutrition Info

Calories 494 Calories from Fat 279

Total Fat 31g 48%

Potassium 1162mg 33%

Total Carbohydrates 12g 4%

Dietary Fiber 5g 20%

Saturated Fat 3g 15%

Cholesterol 93mg 31%

Sodium 83mg 3%

Sugars 4g

Protein 42g 84%

Low Carb Beef Stir Fry

Prep/Cook Time: 20 minutes

Serves: 2

Ingredients:

- ❖ 1 bunch baby bok choy
- ❖ 2 tbs avocado oil or grass-fed ghee, divided
- ❖ 2 tsp coconut aminos
- ❖ 1/4 cup organic broccoli florets
- ❖ 8 oz grass-fed flank
- ❖ 1(One) 1-inch knob of ginger, peeled and cut into thin strips
- ❖ 1/2 cp zucchini, spiralized into 6-inch noodles

Instructions:

- ❖ Cut off your bok choy and discard the end of the stem.
- ❖ Add 1 tablespoon of oil or ghee in a heated pan and sear your steak at medium - high heat on each side for 1-2 minutes.

- ❖ Reduce to medium heat. Add to the pan remaining aminos of ghee, broccoli, ginger and coconut. Cook, stirring frequently, for one minute.
- ❖ Remove choy from bok and cook for another minute.
- ❖ Stir in the zucchini and cook until you prefer the noodles. Watch carefully, because they quickly cook!

Nutrition Info

Calories: 582

Protein: 55g

Carbs: 14g

Fiber: 2g

Sugar: 6g

Net carbs: 12g

Fat: 36g

BBQ Pulled Beef Sando

Prep Time: 8 minutes

Cook Time: 8 hours-12 hours

Total Time: -232 minute

Servings: 4

Ingredients

- 3lbs Boneless Chuck Roast
- 1 tsp onion powder
- 1 tbsp. smoked paprika
- 2 tbsp. tomato paste
- 1/4 cup apple cider vinegar
- 1 tsp black pepper
- 2 tbsp. coconut aminos
- 1/2 cup bone broth
- 2 tsp Pink Himalayan Salt
- 2 tsp garlic powder
- 1/4 cup melted Kerrygold Butter

Instructions

- ❖ Trim the beef fat and slice into two large pieces.
- ❖ Mix salt, garlic, onion, paprika and black pepper in a small bowl. Then rub it over the entire beef. Place the beef in the slow cooker.
- ❖ Melt the butter in another pan, whisk in the amino tomato paste, vinegar and coconut. Verse it over the beef. Then add the slow cooker with the bone broth and pour it around the beef.
- ❖ Set for 10-12 hours on low and cook. Remove the beef when finished, set the slow cooker to high and thicken the sauce. Shred the beef and then add to the slow cooker and cover with the sauce. Serve! Serve!

Nutrition Info

Calories: 184

Fat: 15.1

Carbohydrates: 3.6

Protein: 5.1

Cauliflower Mac and Cheese Recipe & Keto Cheese Sauce

Prep Time: 5 minutes

Cook Time: 20 minutes

Total Time: 25 minutes

Ingredients

- ❖ 1 head Cauliflower (cut into small florets)
- ❖ 3 tbp Butter (divided into 2 tbsp and 1 tbsp)
- ❖ 1/4 cup Heavy cream
- ❖ Sea salt
- ❖ Black pepper
- ❖ 1 cup Cheddar cheese (shredded)
- ❖ 1/4 cp Unsweetened almond milk (or any milk of choice)

Instructions

- ❖ Preheat oven to a temperature of 450 degrees F (232 degrees C). Line a baking sheet of foil or parchment paper.

- ❖ Melt two tablespoons (28 g) of butter. In a large bowl, add the cauliflower flowers to the melted butter. Season with salt and black pepper.
- ❖ Arrange the flowers of the cauliflower on the prepared baking sheet. Roast for about 10-15 minutes, until crisp.
- ❖ Heat cheddar cheese, heavy cream, milk and the remaining spoonful of butter, stirring frequently. (This may be done on the stove as well in a double broiler or in a microwave oven.) Heat until the cheese mixture is smooth. Be careful not to overheat or get the cheese burn.
- ❖ Toss the cauliflower with the cheese sauce just before serving.

Nutrition Info

Calories 294

Fat 23g

Protein 11g

Total Carbs 12g

Net Carbs 7g

Fiber 5g

Sugar 5g

Keto Meatloaf

Prep Time: 10 minutes

Cook Time: 50 minutes

Total Time: 1 hour

Servings: 6

Ingredients

- 1/4 cup chopped fresh oregano
- 4 cloves garlic
- 2 pounds 85% lean grass fed ground beef
- 1/2 tablespoon fine Himalayan salt
- 2 tablespoons avocado oil
- 1 tablespoon lemon zest
- 1/4 cup chopped parsley
- 1 teaspoon black pepper
- 1/4 cup Nutritional Yeast
- 2 large eggs

Instructions

- ❖ Pre-heat 400F oven.
- ❖ The ground beef, black pepper, salt, and nutritional yeast were combined in a large bowl.
- ❖ Mix the eggs, butter, herbs and garlic in a blender or food processor. Stir until the froth is in the eggs and the spices, lemon and garlic are combined.
- ❖ Remove the beef egg blend and mix together.
- ❖ In a thin, 84 loaf pan, add the beef. Quiet and quiet.
- ❖ Place in the oven for 50-60 minutes in the middle rack.
- ❖ Remove the loaf pan from the oven carefully and tip it over the sink to drain the fluid. Let it cool before slicing in for 5-10 minutes.
- ❖ Garnish and enjoy with fresh lemon!

Nutrition Info

Calories: 344

Fat: 29g

Carbohydrates: 4g

Fiber: 2g

Protein: 33g

Caprese Tuna Salad Stuffed Tomatoes

Prep Time: 10 minutes

Servings: Serves 1

Ingredients

- 1 TBSP chopped green onion
- 1 medium tomato
- 1 (5oz) can tuna, very well drained
- 1 TBSP chopped mozzarella {1/4 oz.}
- 1 TBSP chopped fresh basil
- 2 tsp balsamic vinegar

Instructions

- Cut the tomato's top 1/4-inch off. Use a spoon to scoop out the tomato's insides. Set aside as you make the salad for the tuna.
- Mix the drained tuna, balsamic vinegar, mozzarella, basil and green onion together. - the salad of the tuna in the tomato and enjoy it!

❖ Note: I like to use fresh mozzarella, but any mozzarella is good in here.

Nutrition Info

Calories per serving: 196

Fat per serving: 4.9g

Any Time Keto Recipes

Keto Cream Cheese Bread

Keto cream cheese bread is a low-carb recipe made from coconut flour that makes it both keto-friendly and nut-free.

Prep Time: 5 minutes

Cook Time: 25 minutes

Additional Time: 5 minutes

Total Time: 35 minutes

Serving: 12

Ingredients

- ❖ 8 oz of full-fat cream cheese (room temperature)
- ❖ 1 ½ cups coconut flour
- ❖ 1 tablespoon of sugar substitute
- ❖ ½ cup of full-fat sour cream
- ❖ ½ cup of unsalted butter (room temperature)

- 4 teaspoons of baking powder
- 1 teaspoon of sea salt
- 8 large eggs
- 2 tablespoons of sesame seeds (optional)

Instructions

- Allow your eggs to arrive at room temperature, well as cream cheese, butter...
- Preheat the oven to 350 ° C.
- Grease a generously buttered 12-cavity muffin pan or 10-inch loaf pan.
- Add your coconut flour, sea salt, baking powder, sugar substitute and set aside in a medium size dish.
- Beat the room temperature butter together in a large bowl using an electric handheld mixer or a stand-up mixer, cream cheese until light and fluffy. Make sure the bowl sides are scraped multiple times to ensure that the mixture is well blended.

- Combine the 8 eggs one at a time to that butter and cream cheese mixture. Making sure that the sides of the bowl are scratched many times. Note that the mixture will not fully combine due to the large number of eggs, that is normal. After you add the dry ingredients to this wet mix, the ingredients will perfectly blend together.
- In low mixing environment, add all the dry ingredients gradually to the wet ingredients. Make sure the bowl scrapes a few times.
- Once the two mixtures are fully mix stop using the electrical mixture and gently fold in the sour cream 1/2 cup. Make sure that the sour cream is fully incorporated into the batter but be careful not to overmix. Note that the batter is going to be very thick and fluffy. When you are using coconut flour exclusively in a recipe this is the normal texture.
- Just gently overfill the muffin pan. The dense batter won't spread to the muffins. Having

your muffin tins slightly overfilled will create a nice muffin top.

❖ An egg wash is made with one additional whole egg and a spoonful of water. Baste the egg wash at the top of each muffin and sprinkle the sesame seeds over each muffin. That is optional move.

❖ Bake the muffins until lightly brown on top for 25-30 minutes and when an inserted toothpick comes out clean.

❖ Bake the bread for up to 90 mins, if you bake your keto cream cheese bread in a 10 inch loaf. Check your bread for doneness at 60 minutes, and allow longer cooking if needed.

Nutrition Info

Calories: 204 Total Fat: 19.4g Saturated Fat: 11.4g Cholesterol: 154mg Sodium: 160mg Carbohydrates: 2.2g Fiber: 0.6g Sugar: 0.4g Protein: 5.8g

Parmesan & Tomato Keto Bread Buns

Prep Time: 10-15 minutes

Total Time: 55-60 minutes

Ingredients (Makes 5 Buns)

Dry ingredients:

- 1 teasp cream of tartar or apple cider vinegar
- 1/2 teasp baking soda 1/4 cup packed cup flax meal (38 g/ 1.3 ounce)
- 1/3 cp chopped sun-dried tomatoes (37 g/ 1.3 ounce)
- 2/3 cp grated Parmesan cheese (60 g/ 2.1 oz)
- 3/4 (75 g/ 2.7 ounce) cup almond flour
- 2 1/2 (20 g/ 0.7 oz) tablesp psyllium husk powder
- 1/4 cp coconut flour (30 g/ 1.1 ounce)
- 1/4 - 1/2 teasp pink sea salt
- 2 tablesp sesame seeds (18 g/ 0.6 ounce)

Wet ingredients:

- ❖ 1 large egg
- ❖ 1 (240 ml/ 8 fl oz) cups boiling water
- ❖ 3 large egg whites

Instructions

- ❖ Preheat the oven until 175 ° C/ 350 ° F (assisted fan). Use a kitchen scale to weigh all the ingredients and add them to a mixing bowl (apart from the topping sesame seeds): almond flour, coconut flour, flax meal, tartar cream, baking soda, salt, parmesan cheese and sun-dried tomatoes. Mix in all of the dry ingredients. Parmesan & Tomato Keto Bread Buns Add the egg whites and peas, then mix well until the dough is thick.
- ❖ The reason you shouldn't only use whole eggs is because with so many egg yolks in, the buns wouldn't grow. Don't waste them-use them to make Mayo, Quick Hollandaise Sauce or Lemon Curd home made. Parmesan &

Tomato Keto Bread Buns Add boiling water and mix the process until well. Parmesan & Tomato Keto Bread Buns Using a spoon, divide the mixture into 5 keto buns and use your hands to roll into buns. Place them on parchment paper or on a non-stick baking tray. They're going to grow in size, so make sure you leave some room in between. You can use tiny tart trays too.

- ❖ Top each bun with sesame seeds (or any other seeds) and press them gently into the dough, so that they don't fall out. Place in the oven, and cook until golden on top for about 45-50 minutes. Remove from the oven, allow the tray to cool down, and position the buns on a rack to cool to room temperature. Parmesan & Tomato Keto Bread Buns Experience just like regular bread — with butter, bacon, or cheese! Parmesan & Tomato Keto Bread Buns Store for 2-3 days in tupperware, or freeze for up to 3 months.

Note: You Can make 5 regular or large buns as per recipe, or up to 10 small buns.

Nutrition Info

Calories261 kcal

Net carbs4.9 grams

Protein14.5 grams

Fat18.9 grams

15-Minute Gluten Free, Low Carb & Keto Tortillas

This 15-minute gluten-free and keto tortillas are super pliable, quick and make Mexican tacos the best low carb!

Prep Time: 10 minutes

Cook Time: 5 minutes

Total Time: 15 minutes

Servings: 4

Ingredients

- ❖ 1 teaspoon baking powder
- ❖ 1/8-1/4 teaspoon kosher salt depending on whether sweet or savory
- ❖ 96 g almond flour
- ❖ 24 g coconut flour
- ❖ 2 teaspoons xanthan gum
- ❖ 2 teaspoons apple cider vinegar
- ❖ 1 egg lightly beaten
- ❖ 3 teaspoons water

Instructions

- ❖ For food processor add almond flour, coconut flour, xanthan gum, baking powder and salt. Pulse until well combined.
- ❖ Using the food processor, add in apple cider vinegar. When this has been evenly distributed, pour in the egg. The stream followed. Once the dough shapes into a ball, avoid the food processor. The dough is going to get sticky to touch.
- ❖ Wrap the dough in a cling film and knead for a minute or two through the material. Only think of it a little like a ball of heat. Let dough to rest for 10 minutes (and in fridge for up to two days).
- ❖ Heat a skillet over medium heat (preferably), or oven. If the drops evaporate instantly your pan is too dry, you can test the heat by sprinkling a few droplets of water. The droplets should' run' in the skillet.

- ❖ Dissolve the dough into 8 1"balls (26 g each). Roll out with a rolling pin or a tortilla press (easier!) between two sheets of parchment or waxed paper, until each round is 5-inch in diameter.

- ❖ Switch to skillet for just 3-6 seconds and cook over medium heat (very important). Immediately, flip it over (using a thin spatula or knife) and continue to cook for 30 to 40 seconds on each side until just slightly golden (although with traditional charred marks). The trick is not to overcook them, so they won't be pliable or puffed up any more.

- ❖ Keep warm, covered in cooking cloth before serving. Heat briefly on both sides to rewarm, until just warm (less than a minute).

- ❖ Such tortillas are best eaten immediately. Yet feel free to keep up to three days in your fridge to keep some dough handy.

Notes.

Coconut flour burns up rather quickly while cooking. So while this helps you get the traditional charred tortillas marks from flour, you need to keep an eye out for them to keep them from burning. That said, you want your skillet to be very hot, so that the tortillas cook quickly (in less than a minute) and stay pliable. Like any tortilla it will harden and crack if the heat isn't strong enough.

Nutrition Info

Calories 89 Calories from Fat 54

Total Fat 6g 9%

Saturated Fat 1g 5%

Cholesterol 20mg 7%

Sodium 51mg 2%

Potassium 58mg 2%

Total Carbohydrates 4g 1%

Dietary Fiber 2g 8%

Protein 3g 6%

Cheddar Garlic Fathead Rolls

This kind of keto dinner rolls are delicious melt-in-your-mouth. Made from fathead cheddar cheese crust, they are the ideal low carb side dish for all your favorite meals. They even make great sandwiches.

Prep Time 10 mins

Cook Time 25 mins

Total Time 35 mins

Servings: 8 servings

Ingredients

Rolls:

- ❖ 1/4 cp unflavored whey protein powder or may be egg white protein powder
- ❖ 4 teasp baking powder
- ❖ 1 teasp garlic powder
- ❖ 8 oz cheddar cheese grated (I used Cabot Vermont Cheddar)
- ❖ 2 tbsp butter

- ❖ 1/2 cup coconut flour
- ❖ 1/4 tsp salt
- ❖ 2 large eggs
- ❖ 1 large egg white

Garlic Butter

- ❖ 2 tbsp butter melted
- ❖ 2 cloves garlic minced
- ❖ 1 tbsp chopped parsley
- ❖ 1/2 tsp coarse salt

Instructions

- ❖ Preheat the oven to 350F, and line with parchment paper an 8-inch round baking pan.
- ❖ Combine the rubbed cheese and the butter in a big, microwave safe dish. Melt on high in increments of 30 seconds until the cheese and butter can be stirred together and are almost liquid.
- ❖ Add the coconut flour, baking powder, protein powder, salt and garlic powder. In a

bowl, stir in the eggs and egg white and use a rubber spatula to "knead" until even.

❖ Divide the dough into 8 parts which are equal. The dough is going to be pretty sticky so lightly oil your hands and roll into 8 balls. Place in the baking pan to prepare.

❖ Whisk together the garlic butter ingredients, then brush about half of it over the pan rolls.

❖ Bake for at least 20 to 25 minutes, until golden brown, puffed and firm to the touch. Remove and allow to cool for about 15 minutes before removing and breaking apart from pan. Brush with the remaining butter over the garlic. Serving hot.

Nutrition Info

Calories 230 Calories from Fat 143

Total Fat 15.9g 24%

Total Carbohydrates 5.9g 2%

Dietary Fiber 2.6g 10%

Protein 12.2g 24%

Gluten Free, Paleo & Keto Bread

Count on this light, fluffy, absolutely delicious paleo and keto bread with a killer crumb. Plus, this non-eggy sandwich bread will certainly become a favorite, With less than half the amount of eggs as your normal recipe for low carb bread!

Prep Time: 15 minutes

Cook Time: 30 minutes

Resting Time: 40 minutes

Total Time: 45 minutes

Servings: 1

Ingredients

For the paleo & keto bread

- ❖ 1/4 tspoon cream of tartar
- ❖ 1/4 tspoon ground ginger
- ❖ 2 tspoons active dry yeast

- ❖ 2 tspoons maple syrup or honey, to feed the yeast (NO SUGAR WILL BE REMAIN POST BAKE)
- ❖ 120ml water lukewarm between 105-110°F
- ❖ 168g almond flour
- ❖ 83g golden flaxseed meal finely ground
- ❖ 15g whey protein isolate
- ❖ 18g psyllium husk finely ground
- ❖ 2 tspoons xanthan gum or 4 teaspoons ground flaxseed meal**
- ❖ 2 tspoons baking powder
- ❖ 1 tspoon kosher salt
- ❖ 1 egg at room temperature
- ❖ 110g egg whites about 3, at room temperature
- ❖ 56g grass-fed butter or ghee, melted and cooled
- ❖ 1 tblespoon apple cider vinegar
- ❖ 58g sour cream or coconut cream + 2 tsp apple cider vinegar

Instructions

For the paleo & keto bread

- ❖ Fill a loaf pan with 8.5x 4.5 inches of parchment paper (an absolute must!). Set aside.
- ❖ Adding yeast and maple syrup (to feed the yeast into a large bowl. Heat up water to 105-110 ° F and if you do not have a thermometer just feel warm to touch. Pour water over the yeast mixture, cover the bowl with a kitchen towel and let it rest for 7 minutes. If it doesn't start again, the mixture should be bubbly (too cold water doesn't activate the yeast and too hot will destroy it).
- ❖ Mix the flours when proofing the yeast. In a medium bowl, adding the almond flour, flaxseed meal, whey protein powder, psyllium husk, xanthan gum, baking powder, salt, tartar cream and ginger and whisk until thoroughly mixed. Set aside.

❖ Attach egg whites, gently cooled melted butter (you don't want to scramble the eggs or kill the yeast!) and vinegar once the yeast has been confirmed. Mix for a little minutes with an electric mixer, until light and frothy. Put in two lots the flour mixture, alternating with the sour cream, and blend until fully incorporated. To trigger the xanthan gum you want to mix thoroughly and quickly, though the dough will get thick as the flours absorb the moisture.

❖ Move bread dough to prepared loaf pan, using a wet spatula to make the top even out. Cover with a kitchen towel and set for 50-60 minutes in a warm draft-free space until dough has risen just past the top of loaf pan. The length of time it takes depends on your altitude, temperature and humidity, so keep an eye out every 15 minutes. And keep in mind that it won't rise past the top if you are using a larger loaf pan.

- ❖ Preheat oven upto 350 ° F/180 ° C while proofing the dough. And if you bake at high altitude, at 375 ° F/190 ° C you'll want to bake it.
- ❖ Place the loaf saucepan over a baking tray and gently move to the oven. Bake until deep golden for 45-55 minutes and cover with a lose foil dome at minute 10-15 (just as it starts browning). Just be sure the foil doesn't rest directly on the bread.
- ❖ Enable the bread to rest for 5 minutes in the loaf pan, and move it to a cooling rack. Allow for the best texture to cool completely-this is an absolute must, as your keto loaf will continue to cook while it cools! Keep in mind also that a slight deflation is natural, don't sweat it!
- ❖ Hold in an airtight container (or tightly wrapped in a cling film) at room temperature for 4-5 days, before serving, giving it a light toast. Although you will find that even

without toasting this keto bread is surprisingly good!

Note

- If you are paleo (or sustaining keto), feel free to sub 1/4 to 1/2 cup almond flour with arrowroot flour for a lighter crumb.

Nutrition Info

Calories 174 Calories from Fat 126

Total Fat 14g 22%

Saturated Fat 3g 15%

Cholesterol 26mg 9%

Sodium 254mg 11%

Potassium 83mg 2%

Total Carbohydrates 6g 2%

Dietary Fiber 4g 16%

Protein 5g 10%

Keto Mini Bread Loaves

Prep/Cook Time: 1 hour 10 mins

Serving:32

Ingredients

- ❖ 2 tablespoons coconut flour
- ❖ 2 teaspoons Pink Himalayan sea salt
- ❖ 5 teaspoons Apple Cider Vinegar
- ❖ 2 cups almond flour
- ❖ 1/2 cup psyllium husk powder
- ❖ 1/2 cup ground flax
- ❖ 4 teaspoons baking powder
- ❖ 1 3/4 cups boiling water
- ❖ 4 egg whites
- ❖ 2 eggs

Instructions

- ❖ Preheat oven to 350 ° F o.
- ❖ In the medium bowl, mix the almond flour, coconut meal, psyllium husk, flax, sea salt and baking powder.

- ❖ In the meantime, boil the water.
- ❖ Beat the eggs white, eggs, and vinegar lightly in a small bowl (just fast enough to combine all of it).
- ❖ Adding the dry ingredients to the bowl with the eggs and vinegar mixture. Mix for about 20-30 seconds with a hand whisk.
- ❖ Attach the hot water, then whisk 30 seconds more. Then use your hand (be careful, it's still going to be hot), and mix with a folding motion for another 10 seconds. As you do this, the dough will get more "doughy"
- ❖ Since your hands are going to be goopy already, just scoop it into the 4 mini loaf molds equally.
- ❖ Smooth the top a little, but it doesn't have to be flawless.
- ❖ Bake from oven for 50-55 minutes and remove.

- ❖ Lift from loaf pan while they are still dry. To separate the ends, you can use a knife or thin spatula and then pop it out.
- ❖ Let it cool down on the wire rack.

Nutrition Info

Calories 73.28 Total Fat 4.38g Saturated Fat 0.45g Sodium 78.76mg Carbohydrates 6.78g Fiber 4.77g Sugar 0.31g Protein 2.71g

Collagen Keto Bread

Prep/Cook Time: 1 hour and 50 minutes (10 minutes active)

Ingredients:

- ❖ 1/2 cup Unflavored Grass-Fed Collagen Protein
- ❖ 6 tablespoons almond flour
- ❖ Pinch Himalayan pink salt
- ❖ 5 pastured eggs, separated
- ❖ 1 tablespoon unflavored liquid coconut oil
- ❖ 1 teaspoon aluminum-free baking powder
- ❖ 1 teaspoon xanthan gum
- ❖ Optional: pinch of stevia

Instructions:

- ❖ Preheat oven to 325 F.
- ❖ Generously oil with coconut oil (or butter or ghee) only the bottom part of a standard size (1.5quart) glass or ceramic loaf dish. Or you can use a trimmed piece of parchment paper

to match the bottom of your pot. Not oiling or lining your platter's sides will allow the bread to attach to the sides and stay lifted while cooling.

- ❖ Beat the/your egg whites in a large bowl until steep peaks develop. Set aside.
- ❖ Whisk together the dry ingredients in a small bowl and set aside. If you are not a fan of eggs, apply the optional pinch of stevia. Without adding sweetness to your loaf it will help offset the flavor.
- ❖ Whisk the wet ingredients— egg yolks and liquid coconut oil — together in a small bowl, and set aside.
- ❖ To the egg whites, add the dry and wet ingredients and mix until well incorporated. Your batter's going to be a little gooey and heavy.
- ❖ In the oiled or lined dish, pour the batter and place it in the oven.

- ❖ Bake for around 40 minutes. The bread must rise dramatically in the oven.
- ❖ Remove from the oven and let it cool-about 1 to 2 hours. The bread will sink some, and that's fine. Aim the sharp edge of a knife at the sides of the dish once the bread is cooled, to release the loaf.
- ❖ Slice even the slices into 12.
- ❖ Makes: 12 slices

Nutrition Info

Calories: 77

Protein: 7g

Carbs: 1g

Fiber: 1g

Sugar: 0g

Coconut Flour Pizza Crust

This pizza crust made from coconut flour is the best gluten-free pizza crust I've ever tried. It's soft and delicious, and sturdy enough to hold your hands!

Prep Time10 mins

Cook Time20 mins

Total Time30 mins

Servings: 2 (8-inch) pizzas

- ❖ *Ingredients*
- ❖ 1 teaspoon garlic powder
- ❖ 1 teaspoon onion powder
- ❖ 1 teaspoon dried oregano
- ❖ Olive oil spray for pans
- ❖ 4 large eggs
- ❖ 2 tablespoons water
- ❖ 1/4 cup coconut flour
- ❖ 6 tablespoons grated parmesan cheese (1 oz)

Topping:

- ❖ 1/2 cup marinara sauce
- ❖ 1 cup shredded part-skim mozzarella (4 oz)

Instructions

- ❖ Preheat oven to 400 F.
- ❖ Line two parchment paper pizza plates, and dust the paper with olive oil. These pizzas can be made side by side on a single, large baking sheet, too.
- ❖ Whisk the eggs in a large bowl with the water, garlic powder, onion powder and dried orégano.
- ❖ Measure the coconut flour, with your hands breaking up any lumps. In the egg mixture, stir in the coconut flour, mixing until smooth.
- ❖ Whisk in the Parmesan cheese.
- ❖ Allow that mixture to rest for a few minutes, and thicken. This will cause the fluid to soak up from the coconut flour.

- ❖ Use a rubber spatula to transfer half the mixture to each of the prepared panes. Use a spatula to uniformly distribute it over an 8-inch disk.
- ❖ Bake the pizzas until they are set, and the edges start to brown, about 15 minutes. At this level, the crust will still be thin, and that's OK. Remove the pizzas from the oven, and turn the oven to broil. The top oven rack is placed 6 inches below the blaze.
- ❖ Spread half the pizza sauce on each pizza, sprinkle with half the shredded mozzarella and add any other toppings you like (I used pepperoni from Applegate).
- ❖ Broil every pizza for 2-3 minutes until the cheese is melted, and the crust is golden brown.

Nutrition Info

Calories 496 Calories from Fat 297

Total Fat 33g 51%

Saturated Fat 15g 75%

Sodium 885mg 37%

Total Carbohydrates 13g 4%

Dietary Fiber 5g 20%

Sugars 14g

Protein 35g 70%

Gluten Free, Paleo & Keto Drop Biscuits

Ultra-tasty, fast, moist and tender. This paleo and keto drop gluten-free biscuits tick all the right boxes! Whip them up in 30, for an incredibly low carb bread that goes well with both sweet and savory.

Prep Time: 10 minutes

Cook Time: 20 minutes

Total Time: 30 minutes

Servings: biscuits

Ingredients

- ❖ 3 1/2 teaspoons baking powder
- ❖ 1 teaspoon xanthan gum or 1 TBS. flaxseed meal
- ❖ 96g almond flour
- ❖ 63g golden flaxseed meal or psyllium husk, finely ground
- ❖ 21g coconut flour
- ❖ 1 egg

- ❖ 77g sour cream or coconut cream + 2 teasp. apple cider vinegar, at room temp
- ❖ 2 tablespoons water
- ❖ 1 tablespoon apple cider vinegar
- ❖ 20g whey protein isolate or more almond flour
- ❖ 1/2 tspoon kosher salt
- ❖ 112 g organic grass-fed butter or 7 TBS. ghee/coconut oil

Instructions

- ❖ Oven preheat to 450 ° F/230 ° C. Line a parchment paper baking tray, or a baking mat.
- ❖ Inside a medium bowl, add the eggs, sour (or coconut) milk, water and apple cider vinegar then whisk for about a minute or two until fully mixed. Set aside.
- ❖ In a food processor, add almond flour, flaxseed meal, coconut flour, whey protein, baking powder, xanthan gum (or more flax), and kosher salt and pulse until very thoroughly combined.

- ❖ Add in the butter and pump until pea-sized a few times. Pour in the mixture of the egg and cream, pulsing until mixed. The dough is going to be quite shaggy.
- ❖ Drop the dough 6 rounds onto the prepared baking tray. Brush with melted butter and bake until deep golden for 15-20 minutes. Before serving allow to cool for 10 minutes. These guys stay well, kept at room temperature in an airtight container for 3-4 days.
- ❖ The shaped biscuit dough can be frozen for 1-2 months, and baken directly from the freezer as required.

Nutrition Info

Calories 290 Calories from Fat 270

Total Fat 30g 46%

Saturated Fat 11g 55%

Cholesterol 74mg 25%

Sodium 455mg 19%

Potassium 113mg 3%

Total Carbohydrates 8g 3%

Dietary Fiber 5g 20%

Sugars 1g

Protein 7g 14%

Low Carb Bagels-Gluten Free Onion Sesame

Prep/Cook Time: 20 mins

Servings: 4

Ingredients

- 3 eggs
- 1 1/2 cups almond flour
- 1 Tablespoon onion powder
- 2 1/2 cups mozzerella cheese
- 2 ounces cream cheese
- 1/2 teaspoon salt
- 1 Tablespoon sesame seeds

Instructions

- Preheat oven to 400 F.
- Mozzarella cheese and cream cheese melt together over a double boiler.
- Stir and beat in 2 eggs, when melted.
- Add almond flour, onion powder, and salt, in a separate bowl. Stir to combine.

- ❖ Pour the flour mixture into a mixture of cheese / egg and blend well.
- ❖ Take a small handful (about the size of an orange) and shape into a ball, using wet hands. Flap and make a hole in the middle.
- ❖ Lay the bagels on a baking sheet lined with parchment.
- ❖ Beat the rest of the egg, and brush over the bagels.
- ❖ Sprinkle the bagels with sesame seeds and put them in the oven. Bake until golden brown, for 12 minutes. Remove the baking sheet, and allow it to cool.

Nutrition Info

Calories: 287 Total Fat: 23g Unsaturated Fat: 14g Cholesterol: 105mg Sodium: 401mg Saturated Fat: 7g Trans Fat: 0g Carbohydrates: 7g Fiber: 3g Sugar: 2g Protein: 15g

Cranberry Jalapeño "Cornbread" Muffins

Low carb, muffins which taste like cornbread! These delicious muffins, made from coconut flour and bursting with cranberries and jalapeño, would make a great addition to any Thanksgiving table.

Prep Time 10 mins

Cook Time 30 mins

Total Time 40 mins

Servings: 12 muffins

Calories: 157 kcal

Ingredients

- ❖ 7 large eggs, lightly beaten
- ❖ 1 cup unsweetened almond milk
- ❖ 1/2 cup butter, melted OR avocado oil
- ❖ 1 cup coconut flour (I used Bob's Red Mill)
- ❖ 1/3 cup Swerve Sweetener or other erythritol
- ❖ 1 tbsp baking powder

- ❖ 1/2 tsp salt
- ❖ 1/2 tsp vanilla
- ❖ 1 cup fresh cranberries, cut in half
- ❖ 3 tbsp minced jalapeño peppers
- ❖ 1 jalapeño, seeds removed, sliced into 12 slices, for garnish

Instructions

- ❖ Preheat oven to 325F and grate well or line with paper liners on a muffin tin.
- ❖ Whisk the coconut flour, sweetener, baking powder and salt together in a medium bowl. Split some clumps with a fork backside.
- ❖ Add the eggs, butter and almond milk melted, and whisk vigorously. Add the vanilla extract and continue stirring until the mixture is smooth and combined well. Stir in chopped jalapeños and cranberries.
- ❖ Divide batter equally between prepared cups of muffins and put one slice of jalapeño on top of each one.

❖ Bake for 25 minutes to 30 minutes or until tops are set, and a centered tester comes out clean. Let it cool down in pan for 10 minutes, then move to a wire rack to completely cool.

Nutrition Info

Calories 157 Calories from Fat 101

Total Fat 11.22g 17%

Saturated Fat 7.11g 36%

Cholesterol 128mg 43%

Sodium 362mg 15%

Total Carbohydrates 7.08g 2%

Dietary Fiber 3.84g 15%

Protein 5.21g 10%

Paleo Chocolate Zucchini Bread

Paleo Chocolate Bread with Zucchini. Healthy, natural gluten free, super moist with almond meal and cocoa powder that is not sweetened. 100% KETO + low carb + free sugar

Prep Time10 mins

Cook Time50 mins

Cool down4 hrs

Total Time1 hr

Servings: 12 slices

Calories: 185kcal

Ingredients

Dry ingredients

- ❖ 2 teaspoons ground cinnamon
- ❖ 1/4 teaspoon sea salt
- ❖ 1 1/2 cup almond flour (170g)
- ❖ 1/4 cup unsweetened cocoa powder (25g)

- ❖ 1 1/2 teaspoon baking soda
- ❖ 1/2 cup sugar free crystal sweetener (Monk fruit or erythritol) (100g) or coconut sugar if refined sugar free

Wet ingredients

- ❖ 1/4 cup + 2 tablespoon canned coconut cream 100ml
- ❖ 1/4 cp extra virgin coconut oil , melted, 60ml
- ❖ 1 cup zucchini, finely grated measure packed, discard juice/liquid if there is some - about 2 small zucchini
- ❖ 1 large egg
- ❖ 1 teaspoon vanilla extract
- ❖ 1 teaspoon apple cider vinegar

Filling - optional

- ❖ 1/2 cup sugar free chocolate chips
- ❖ 1/2 cp chopped walnuts or any other nuts you like

Instructions

- ❖ Preheat oven until 375F (180C). Line a baking loaf pan with parchment paper (9"x 5"). Set aside.
- ❖ Remove both ends of the zucchinis, just leave the skin on.
- ❖ Using a vegetable grater finely brush the zucchini. Measure the required amount in a measuring cup. Make sure you press / pack them firmly for a precise measure and I usually do not have any! to squeeze out any liquid from the grated zucchini. If you do, dump or hold the liquid for another recycle.
- ❖ In a large mixing bowl, stir all of the dry ingredients together: almond flour, unsweetened cocoa powder, sugar-free crystal sweetener, cinnamon, sea salt and baking soda. Set aside.
- ❖ In the dry ingredients, add all the wet ingredients: grated courgettes, coconut oil,

coconut cream, cinnamon, sugar, apple cider vinegar.

- ❖ Stir both ingredients together to blend.
- ❖ Stir in the chopped chocolate chips and sugar free nuts.
- ❖ Move the batter of chocolate bread into the prepared loaf pan.
- ❖ Bake 50-55 minutes, maybe after 40 minutes you want to cover the bread loaf with a piece of foil to avoid darkening the top too much, up to you.
- ❖ Upon completely cooling down, the bread should remain slightly moist in the center and firm up.

Cool Down

- ❖ Cool down in the loaf pan for 10 minutes, then cool down on a refrigerating rack until it reaches room temperature. It can take four hours, because it's a thick bread. Don't slice the bread until it reaches room temperature. If it's too hot in the centre, when you slice it will be too often and fall apart. Cool down at room temperature for 40 minutes then pop in the refrigerator for 1 hour for a faster result. The fridge will create an extra fudgy texture, making it even easier to slice the bread as it firms up.

❖ Store in a cake bow or airtight container in the refrigerator for up to 4 days.

Nutrition Info

Calories: 185kcal, Carbohydrates: 6.1g, Protein: 4.9g, Fat: 17.1g, Fiber: 2.7g, Sugar: 1.2g

Garlic, Dill & Cheddar Keto Bread

Prep/Cook Time: 55 minutes

Ingredients

- ¼ teaspoon kosher salt (1.2 ml)
- 3 teaspoons aluminum-free baking powder (15 ml)
- ¼ teaspoon cream of tartar (1.2 ml)
- 1 ½ cps blanched almond flour (165 g)
- 4 large eggs, separated
- 1 tblespoon egg white protein powder (5 g)
- 5 tblespoons unsalted butter, melted and cooled (70 g)
- 1 teaspoon garlic powder (5 ml)
- 1 teaspoon dried dill (5 ml)
- 1 cup grated cheddar cheese (90g)

Instructions

- Preheat oven to F/190o C, 375o.

- ❖ Fill a 8.5x 4.5 loaf pan with light grease. Cover the bottom side of the loaf pan with finely grated parchment paper for easiest release.
- ❖ The almond flour, egg yolks, egg white protein powder, butter, salt and baking powder are combined in a food processor.
- ❖ If cinnamon & honey bread is been made, add the cinnamon and honey.
- ❖ When making bread with garlic, dill & cheddar, add the garlic powder, dill and cheddar.
- ❖ Just process until the ingredients come together in a dough ball.
- ❖ Combine the egg whites and tartar cream into the bowl of an electric mixer. Using the whisk attachment, whisk until the egg whites are large and fluffy and form soft peaks (when the whisk is lifted from the egg whites, it should form a soft peak, then fall slightly).
- ❖ Pour one-third of the egg whites into the food processor. Pulse till combined, scrap the sides

as needed. Attach another 1/3 of the egg whites and pump into a wet batter again until mixed.

Primal.

- ❖ With the remaining egg whites, scrape the dough out of the food processor into the cup. Using a spatula to fold the egg whites gently into the dough. Gently fold and mix until there are no white streaks, but be gentle; the air in the whites of the egg helps the dough to rise to a light textured loaf.
- ❖ Scrape the loaf batter into the pan. Bake in for 30 minutes.
- ❖ Let cool off from the loaf pan for at least 30 minutes before removing. Seek to let the loaf cool before slicing down completely on a wire rack.
- ❖ Primal keto bread is placed on the counter for 1 to 2 days, simply with a thin towel above it. Hold the keto bread tightly wrapped in a towel

inside a sealed plastic bag in the refrigerator for longer storage (3 to 5 days).

Recipe Notes.

If the baking powder is aluminum-free (usually on the front of the can), the baked goods will not have a strange metallic flavour. Another possible reason to use aluminum-free: Baking aluminum powder will give a grayish color to baked goods if acidic ingredient is included in the recipe.

Jenni Treesong

Cauliflower Bread Recipe with Garlic & Herbs

This cauliflower garlic & herb bread loaf makes a healthy & delicious keto, paleo, low carb garlic bread! Ideal also for low-carb sandwiches.

Prep Time 15 minutes

Cook Time 45 minutes

Total Time 1 hour

Ingredients

- ❖ 6 tablesp Butter (measured solid, unsalted, then melted; can use ghee for dairy-free)
- ❖ 6 cloves Garlic (minced)
- ❖ 1 1/4 cup Coconut flour
- ❖ 1 1/2 tbsp Gluten-free baking powder
- ❖ 1 tsp Sea salt
- ❖ 3 cup Cauliflower ("riced" using food processor*)
- ❖ 10 large Egg (separated)
- ❖ 1/4 tsp Cream of tartar (optional)

- ❖ 1 tbsp Fresh rosemary (chopped)
- ❖ 1 tbsp Fresh parsley (chopped)

Instructions

- ❖ Oven preheat to 350 degrees F (177 degrees C). Line a 9x5 in (23x13 cm) parchment-paper loaf pan.
- ❖ The riced cauliflower is steamed. You can do this in a microwave (cooked for 3-4 minutes, lined with plastic) OR in a steamer basket over the water on the stove (line with cheesecloth if the steamer basket holes are too large, and steam for a few minutes). Both ways, steam soft and tender until the cauliflower is soft. Let cool enough for the cauliflower to handle
- ❖ In the meantime, beat the egg whites and tartar cream with a hand mixer until stiff peaks form.
- ❖ In a food processor put the coconut flour, baking powder, melted butter, sea salt, egg yolks, 1/4 whipped egg whites and garlic.

- ❖ When the cauliflower has cooled enough to treat, wrap it in a kitchen towel and press as many times as possible to absorb as much moisture. (This is important-the end result should be very dry and clump together.) Add the food processor to the cauliflower. Combined process until well. (The mixture is thick and somewhat crumbly.) Adding the remaining egg whites to the food processor. Fold in just a bit, to make the loading simpler. Pulse until it has just been implemented a few times. Fold in chopped parsley and rosemary. (The mixture will be fluffy.) (Do not overmix the egg whites too much to avoid breaking down.) Move the batter to the lined baking pan. Smooth the top, and slightly round. You can press more herbs to the top if needed (optional).
- ❖ Bake for about 45-50 minutes, until golden is on top. Before removing and slicing, completely Cool.

- ❖ Making Buttered Low Carb Garlic Bread (optional): Top slices generously with butter, sliced garlic, fresh parsley, and some salt from the sea. Bake for about 10 mins in a preheated oven, at 450 degrees F (233 degrees C). Put/place under the broiler for a few minutes, if you want to brown it more.

Nutrition Info

Calories 108

Fat 8g

Protein 6g

Total Carbs 8g

Net Carbs 3g

Fiber 5g

Sugar 3g

Keto Bagel Recipe

Are you missing a good bagel in your Keto lifestyle? Now you don't have to!

Prep Time: 5 minutes

Cook Time: 25 minutes

Serving: 2

Ingredients

- ❖ 1 teaspoon (2 g) of baking powder
- ❖ 2 1/2 Tbspoons (38 ml) of ghee, melted
- ❖ 1 Tbspoon (15 ml) of olive oil
- ❖ 1 teaspoon (3 g) of garlic powder
- ❖ pinch salt
- ❖ 1 cup (120 g) of almond flour
- ❖ 1/4 cup coconut flour (28 g)
- ❖ 1 Tbspoon (7 g) of psyllium husk powder
- ❖ 2 medium eggs (88 g)
- ❖ 2 tspoons (10 ml) of white wine vinegar
- ❖ 1 teaspoon (5 g) of sesame seeds

Instructions

- ❖ Oven preheat to 160 ° C (320 ° F).
- ❖ Combine in a bowl the almond flour, coconut flour, baking powder, psyllium husk powder, garlic powder and salt.
- ❖ Whisk the eggs together and the vinegar in a separate bowl. Drizzle slowly in the melted ghee (which shouldn't pip hot) and whisk in well.
- ❖ Apply the wet mixture to the dry mixture, and blend well using a wooden spoon. Exit for 2-3 minutes to sit down.
- ❖ Divide the mixture into 4 portions of the same size. Shape the mixture into a round shape using your hands, and put it on a tray lined with parchment paper. Using a small spoon or apple corer to create a hole in the centre.
- ❖ Brush with olive oil to the tops and scatter over the seeds of sesame. Bake 20-25 minutes in the

oven until cooked. Allow to cool down before enjoying yourself!

Nutrition Info

Calories: 629 Carbohydrates: 19 g Sugar: 4 g Fat: 56 g Fiber: 12 g Protein: 19 g

Keto Pull Apart Clover Rolls

Keto Pull Apart Clover Rolls is the best low carb gluten-free wheels I've ever made! Soft, buttery, cheesy rolls pulling apart like a three-leaf clover into three sections

Prep Time 7 mins

Cook Time 20 mins

Total Time 27 mins

Servings:4

Ingredients

- ❖ 1 ½ tsp baking powder
- ❖ 1 ½ cup shredded Mozzarella cheese
- ❖ 2 ounces cream cheese
- ❖ 1 ½ cup blanched almond flour or can also use 1/3 cup coconut flour instead
- ❖ ¼ cup grated Parmesan cheese
- ❖ 2 lg eggs

Instructions

- ❖ Grease or spray a muffin pan with the non-stick oil and preheat the oven to 350 F.
- ❖ Combine the almond flour & baking powder in a mixing bowl, then blend well. Set aside.
- ❖ Melt the shredded Mozzarella as well as the cream cheese over the top of the stove (or 1 minute in the microwave) until melted.
- ❖ Once the cheese has melted, add eggs and flour blend. Mix together.
- ❖ Knead the hands and knead the dough into a sticky ball. Place the ball of dough on a large sheet of baking paper or on a silicone mat.
- ❖ Slice a ball of dough into fourths. Slice then into 6 small pieces each fifth.
- ❖ Form the small pieces into balls, and form the balls gently in a Parmesan cheese bowl to cover them slightly with Parmesan (this allows them to quickly fall apart).

- ❖ In the muffin pan, add 3 of the dough balls to each muffin cup (that makes the 3 leaf clover).
- ❖ Bake for 20 minutes at 350 F, or until golden brown. Remove from the oven before serving and allow to cool slightly.

Nutrition Info

Calories 283 Calories from Fat 189

Total Fat 21g 32%

Saturated Fat 8g 40%

Total Carbohydrates 6g 2%

Dietary Fiber 2g 8%

Sugars 1g

Protein 16g 32%

Keto Flax Seed Bread

Prep Time 5 minutes

Cook Time 2 minutes

Total Time 7 minutes

Servings 2 Slices

Ingredients

- ❖ 1 tablespoon Softened Butter
- ❖ 4 tablespoons Organic Ground Flaxseed Meal
- ❖ 1 Large Egg
- ❖ ½ teaspoon Baking Powder
- ❖ ½ teaspoon Salt

Instructions

- ❖ Take your square Pyrex glass dish and add the butter. In the microwave melt for a few seconds.
- ❖ Crack the egg into the bowl, and blend well with a fork.

- In another bowl, mix the ground flax seed, salt and baking powder, and blend.
- Adding all mixed dry ingredients, ground flax, salt, and baking powder to the baking dish and thoroughly blend all ingredients.
- It will turn into a dense layer. To ensure even cooking, flatten out the surface of the mixture.
- Two minutes in the microwave to cook.
- Until taking out, leave to cool for a few minutes.
- Use a spatula and pull the bread gently off the side of the platter. It should come out without any trouble after you turn it upside down.
- Take your knife and cut it half way to make two slices

3 Minute Low Carb Biscuits

Prep Time: 2 minutes

Cook Time: 3 minutes

Total Time: 5 minutes

Servings: 1 Servings

Calories: 392kcal

Ingredients

- 1/4 cup Cheddar Cheese
- 1/8 tsp garlic powder
- 1/8 tsp Onion powder
- 1/8 tsp Dried Parsley
- 1 tbsp Butter
- 2 tbsp Coconut flour
- 1 large Egg
- 1 tbsp Heavy Whipping Cream
- 2 tbsp Water
- 1/8 tsp Pink Himalayan Salt
- 1/8 tsp black pepper

- ❖ 1/4 tsp Baking powder

Instructions

- ❖ Melt butter for 20 seconds in a coffee mug by microwaving.
- ❖ Add the flour with coconut, baking powder and seasonings. Combine with a fork to add.
- ❖ Add the heavy whipping cream, egg, and cheese. Mix until blend.
- ❖ Microwave for three minutes. Remove from mug immediately and allow to cool down for 2 minutes.
- ❖ Slice, and have fun.

Nutrition Info

Calories: 392kcal, Carbohydrates: 9g, Protein: 15g, Fat: 32g, Fiber: 5g

Coconut Flour Psyllium Husk Bread - Paleo

Are you looking to have an easy low carb keto Paleo bread? Try this recipe for gluten-free psyllium bread in coconut flour. Breakfast or dinner is a tasty bread to serve.

Prep Time 5 minutes

Cook Time 55 minutes

Total Time 1 hour

Servings 15 slices

Calories 127kcal

Ingredients

- ❖ 6 tablespoons whole psyllium husks 27g, may want to finely grind
- ❖ 3/4 cup warm water
- ❖ 1 cup coconut flour 125g
- ❖ 1 1/2 teaspoons baking soda
- ❖ 3/4 teaspoon sea salt

- ❖ 1 pint egg whites 2 cups (or use 8 whole eggs)
- ❖ 2 large eggs
- ❖ 1/2 cup olive oil
- ❖ 1/4 cup coconut oil melted

Instructions

- ❖ Preheat oven to 350 degrees F.
- ❖ If not to use silicone pan, grease pan or line pan with parchment paper. I used that 8x4-in pan.
- ❖ Dump all ingredients and pulse until well mixed into a food processor. If you do not have a food processor you can use an electric mixer mixing cup.
- ❖ Spread batter into loaf pan with 8x4. Smooth top.
- ❖ Bake for 45-55 minutes or until brown edges are inserted and clean the toothpick.
- ❖ Let the bread sit for 15 minutes in a saucepan. Remove the bread from the saucepan and allow the rack to cool.

Notes

Original recipe used an egg carton that may give rise to an odor of ammonia. The recipe has therefore changed to 1 pint egg whites and 2 whole eggs.

Nutrition Info

Calories 127 Calories from Fat 120

Total Fat 13.3g 20%

Sodium 243mg 10%

Total Carbohydrates 6g 2%

Dietary Fiber 4.1g 16%

Protein 3g 6%

Homemade Nut and Seed Paleo Bread

Prep Time: 10 min

Cook Time: 40 min

Total Time: 50 minutes

Serving: 12 -15 slices

Ingredients

- 1/4 cup chia meal (just blender or grind chia seed in a coffee grinder) or use ground flaxseed
- Pumpkin seed for topping and Extra poppyseed
- 1/2 teasp sea salt
- dash of black pepper
- Optional 1 teasp spice mix of choice (garlic, rosemary, Italian, etc.).
- 1 – 2 teasp poppyseed (plus extra for topping)
- 1 1/4 cup almond flour
- 5 eggs (6 if you want more fluffy)
- 1/3 cup coconut oil or avocado oil

- 1 teasp white vinegar or apple cider vinegar
- 3 to 4 tablesp tapioca flour (if you are using more egg, add 4 tbsp).
- 1/2 tsp baking soda

Instructions

- Preheat oven until 350. Grease a parchment paper pan or line of 9 x 5 breadpan. Set aside. Use an 8⁄4 pan for higher higher bread.
- Whisk your eggs, butter, and vinegar in a small saucepan.
- Combine the flours, poppyzeed and seasonings in another tub.
- Attach your wet ingredients and blend well to dry ingredients.
- Pour batter into greased pan and cover with additional and poppyseed pumpkin seeds.
- Covered Bake for 20 minutes. Then uncover and continue baking for 15-20 more or golden and clean knife in the center.

- ❖ Depending on your oven, should all be about 35-45 minutes together. If you used 8 x 4 or baked higher, you may need to bake longer.
- ❖ Clear from the frying pan and let cool.
- ❖ Wrap, slice and store the paleo bread in foil or plastic wrap. Keeps well in refrigerator for up to seven days or freezer for up to three months.

Notes

If you're looking for a vegan or egg-free option you can try to replace the eggs with 3/4 cup aquafaba. It bakes but not much rises. All yummy!

Low Carb Pumpkin Bread

Prep Time: 15 minutes

Cook Time: 45 minutes

Total Time: 1 hour

Serving: 20

Ingredients

- ❖ 15 oz. can of pumpkin puree
- ❖ 2 cups granulated of sugar substitute
- ❖ 3 teaspoons of baking powder
- ❖ 2 teaspoon vanilla extract
- ❖ 3 tablespoons of pumpkin pie spice
- ❖ 3 tablespoons of cinnamon powder
- ❖ 1/4 teaspoon sea salt
- ❖ 10 large eggs
- ❖ 3 cups of almond flour
- ❖ 1 cup of golden flax meal
- ❖ Optional
- ❖ Cream Cheese Frosting
- ❖ 8 oz package of softened cream cheese

- 4 tablespoons of heavy whipping cream
- 1 cup of sugar-free confectioners sugar

Instructions

- Preheat the oven to 350 ° C.
- Grease two loaf pans 8x4 inches well.
- Beat the pumpkin puree, sugar substitute, and vanilla extract with an electric mixer until it is well blended.
- Then add one at a time in the eggs to make sure that they beat before completely combined.
- Add the almond flour and flax seed, baking powder, spices and salt to the wet batter.
- Remember batter is going to be thick Pour the batter into the two pans and bake for 45 mins at 350 degrees, or until an inserted toothpick comes out clean.

Notes

This recipe makes two large loaves of low carb pumpkin bread and froze well.

Nutrition Info

Calories: 200 Total Fat: 15.8g Saturated Fat: 5.5g Cholesterol: 59mg Sodium: 60mg Carbohydrates: 4.8g Fiber: 2.9g Sugar: 0.8g Protein: 6.4g

Cheesy Skillet Bread

Easy low carb skillet bread with a sumptuous cheddar cheese crust. This recipe for keto bread is good for soups and stews, and makes the BEST low carb Thanksgiving stuffing!

Prep Time 10 mins

Cook Time 16 mins

Total Time 26 mins

Servings: 10

Ingredients

- ❖ 1 tbsp butter for the skillet
- ❖ 2 cups almond flour
- ❖ 1/2 cup flax seed meal
- ❖ 2 tsp baking powder
- ❖ 1/2 tsp salt
- ❖ 1 1/2 cps shredded Cheddar cheese divided
- ❖ 3 large eggs lightly beaen
- ❖ 1/2 cup butter melted

- ❖ 3/4 cup almond milk

Instructions

- ❖ Oven preheat to 425F. Fill a 10-inch oven-proof skillet with 1 tbsp of butter and put in the oven.
- ❖ Whisk the almond flour, flax seed meal, baking powder, salt and 1 cup shredded cheddar cheese together in a large bowl.
- ❖ Adding the eggs, melted butter, and almond milk until well combined.
- ❖ Remove the hot skillet from the oven (remember to put the mitts on your pan), and swirl the butter to the side of the brush.
- ❖ Pour batter into a casserole and smooth the top. Sprinkle with 1/2 cup remaining cheddar.
- ❖ Bake for 16 minutes to 20 minutes, or until browned around the edges and set midway through. Cheese should be well browned up on top.
- ❖ Remove, then allow it to cool for 15 minutes.

Recipe Notes

Serves 10. Each serving has 7.2 g of carbs & 4 g of fiber. Total NET CARBS = 3.2 g.

Nutrition Info

Calories 357 Calories from Fat 276

Total Fat 30.63g 47%

Total Carbohydrates 7.9g 3%

Dietary Fiber 4.77g 19%

Protein 12.48g 25%

Turmeric Cauliflower Buns

This 4-Ingredient Turmeric Cauliflower Buns are an easy side dish that is grain-free, low-carb and super healthy.

Prep Time: 30 mins

Cook Time: 30 mins

Serving: 6

Ingredients

- ❖ 2 eggs
- ❖ 2 tablespoons coconut flour
- ❖ 1 medium head of cauliflower or about 2 cups of firmly packed cauliflower rice
- ❖ ¼ teaspoon ground turmeric
- ❖ pinch each of salt and pepper

Instructions

- ❖ Oven preheat to 400 ° F.
- ❖ Line a parchment-papered baking sheet and set aside.

❖ Take your cauliflower and cut off the base with a sharp knife. Use your hands to split the cauliflower into florets and pick off any green parts. Give quick rinse and pat dry to the florets.

❖ Next, make cauliflower rice by putting the florets with the "S" blade in a food processor's bowl. Pulse until the cauliflower is about or almost the size of the rice for about 30 seconds. You should have about two cups of cauliflower rice that is firmly packed.

❖ Layer the cauliflower rice with around a teaspoon of water in a microwave-safe cup. Cover with plastic wrap and poke a couple of holes to let the steam run away. Microwave around 3 minutes of the cauliflower rice. Instead, the cauliflower rice can be steamed in a steamer basket on the stovetop.

❖ Uncover the bowl and allow about 5 minutes to cool the cauliflower rice. Then put the cauliflower rice in a nut milk bag or a clean dish towel with a large spoon. Extra moisture squeeze out, be careful not to burn your palms.

❖ In a small mixing bowl, add the cauliflower rice and stir in the eggs, turmeric and a pinch of salt and black pepper.

❖ Use your hands to shape the blend into 6 buns and put them on the baking sheet.

❖ Bake for 25-30 minutes, or until slightly browning on top.

❖ The cauliflower buns are best served directly from the oven, soft. They don't cool or heat well (they're going to get mushy), but they're so delicious that you're going to eat them immediately!

Nutrition Info

Calories Per Serving: 59

% Daily Value

3% Total Fat 2.1g

21% Cholesterol 62mg

6% Sodium 151.7mg

2% Total Carbohydrate 6.6g

Sugars 2.4g

9% Protein 4.5g

2% Vitamin A 26.7μg

79% Vitamin C 47.2mg

3% Calcium 31.2mg

4% Magnesium 17mg

Buttery Low Carb Flatbread

The best from the sliced bread. Mostly because it is gluten-free, fried and in butter slathered.

Prep time 5 mins

Cook time 2 mins

Total time 7 mins

Serves: 4

Ingredients

- ❖ 1 tbsp Oil for frying
- ❖ 1 tbsp melted Butter-for slathering
- ❖ 1 cup Almond Flour
- ❖ 2 tbsp Coconut Flour
- ❖ 2 tsp Xanthan Gum
- ❖ ½ tsp Baking Powder
- ❖ ½ tsp Falk Salt + more to garnish
- ❖ 1 Whole Egg + 1 Egg White
- ❖ 1 tbsp Water

Instructions

- ❖ Whisk the dry ingredients together (flours, xanthan gum, baking powder, salt) until well blended.
- ❖ Add the white egg and egg and gently beat for incorporation into the flour. The dough is about to start forming.
- ❖ Attach the tablespoon of water and start working the dough to allow the moisture to absorb the flour and xanthan gum.
- ❖ Cut the dough into 4 (four) equal parts and press out each segment with a fastener.
- ❖ Heat over medium heat a large skillet, and add oil.
- ❖ Fry each flat-bread on each side for about 1 min.
- ❖ Sprinkle with butter (when warm) and garnish with salt and chopped parsley.
- ❖ Just split the dough into 5 balls instead of 4, if you want a smaller portion!

Nutrition Info

Serving size: 1 flatbread Calories: 232 Fat: 19 Carbohydrates: 9 Fiber: 5 Protein: 9

Paleo Gluten-Free Low Carb English Muffin

A paleo low carb English muffin recipe which is soft and buttery inside, crusty on the outside. This gluten-free English muffins are easy to make with 5 ingredients in 2 minutes!

Prep Time 2 minutes

Cook Time 3 minutes

Total Time 5 minutes

Ingredients

- ❖ 1 pinch Sea salt
- ❖ 1/2 tsp Gluten-free baking powder
- ❖ 1 large Egg (or equivalent egg whites)
- ❖ 3 tbsp Blanched almond flour
- ❖ 1/2 tbsp Coconut flour
- ❖ 1 tablesp Butter (or ghee, or coconut oil)

Instructions

- ❖ Melt ghee (or butter) in a ramekin or other container that is safe for microwaves or ovens, about 4 in (10 cm) diameter with a flat base. It takes about 30 seconds to do so. (If you only use an oven, melt it in the oven while it is preheating. Remove once melted.) Adding the remaining ingredients and stir until well mixed. Let sit for a minute, to thicken the mixture.
- ❖ Microwave Method: Microwave until firm for about 90 seconds.
- ❖ Oven method: Bake at 350 degrees F (177 degrees C) for about 15 minutes, until the top is firm and spring-y to the touch.
- ❖ Travel along the edge of a knife and flip over a plate to release. In the toaster, slice in half, then toast.

Recipe Notes

If you want more / smaller slices, instead of a ramekin, you can also make it in a mug, then just pop those in the toaster in batch.

Serving size: 2 large slices (entire recipe)

Nutrition Info

Calories 307

Fat 27g

Protein 12g

Total Carbs 8g

Net Carbs 4g

Fiber 4g

Sugar 2g

Cauliflower Tortillas

Great low carb alternative to traditional flour tortillas or corn.

Prep Time 30 minutes

Cook Time 20 minutes

Total Time 50 minutes

Servings 6 tortillas

Calories 37

Ingredients

- ❖ 1/2 medium lime, juiced and zested
- ❖ salt & pepper, to taste
- ❖ 3/4 large head cauliflower (or two cups riced)
- ❖ 2 large eggs (Vegans, sub flax eggs)
- ❖ 1/4 cup chopped fresh cilantro

Instructions

- ❖ Preheat an/the oven to 375 degrees F., and line the baking sheet with parchment paper.

- ❖ Trim the cauliflower, cut it into small, uniform pieces and pulse in batches in a food processor until you get a consistency similar to a couscous. The finely riced cauliflower should be packed into about 2 cups.
- ❖ Place the coliflower for 2 minutes in a microwave-safe bowl and microwave, then stir again and microwave for another 2 minutes. If you're not using a microwave, then a steamer works just as well. Put the cauliflower in a fine cheesecloth or thin dishtowel, squeeze out as much liquid as possible, making sure you don't burn. Gloves are suggested for dishwashing, as it is very hot.
- ❖ Whisk the eggs into a medium bowl. Add cauliflower, coriander, lime, salt and pepper to taste. Blend well until combined. Use your hands on the parchment paper to shape 6 small "tortillas"
- ❖ Bake for 10 minutes, flip each tortilla carefully, and then return to the oven for

another 5 to 7 minutes or until completely set. Place tortillas on a wire rack to slightly cool off.

❖ Heat on a medium sized skillet. Place a baked tortilla into the oven, slightly press down and brown on each side for 1 to 2 minutes. Repeat with tortillas left on.

Keto Fiber Bread Rolls Recipe

These Low Carb and Keto Fiber Bread Rolls Recipe are made perfectly and are extremely delicious and irresistible to make. One look at them will persuade you to try and get them right at this moment.

Prep Time 10 minutes

Cook Time 40 minutes

Total Time 50 minutes

Serving: 11 Serving Size: 1

Ingredients

- 15g (3Tbsp)Psyllium Husk
- 250g (1 Cup)Greek Yogurt
- 4 Eggs
- 150g (1.5 Cups) Almond Flour
- 30g (1/4 Cup) Protein
- 1 Pkt (16g)(4tsp) Baking Powder
- 75g (3/4 Cup)Potato or Oat Fiber
- 4 Tbsp (25g) Oil

- ❖ 2 Tbsp Water
- ❖ 2 Tbsp Vinegar
- ❖ 1 tsp salt

Instructions

- ❖ Heat the oven until 150C or 300F.
- ❖ Blend dry ingredients together.
- ❖ Separate eggs, and first mix all the egg whites. Deposit aside.
- ❖ Mix well, the egg yolks.
- ❖ Stir in yogurt and all the wet ingredients.
- ❖ Keep adding all the combined dry ingredients spoon by spoon.
- ❖ Add egg whites at the end and gently and blend properly.
- ❖ Cover the bowl for half an hour, and let it rest.
- ❖ Prepare a sheet of Parchment paper for baking.
- ❖ When relaxed, make small balls with wet side, which you then flatten with hands to create rolls a bit at the end.

- ❖ Once everything is on the baking sheet, add a bit of Potato or Oat Fiber to obtain the white look after baking.
- ❖ With your super Kaiser Roll Shaper Gadget knife, press each Roll to give it the perfect finishing touch.
- ❖ Place in the oven and bake 40 Minutes.
- ❖ Bon Appetit.

Notes. Notes.

You can use Potato Fiber or Oat Fiber for this recipe to achieve the results which are the same.

Nutrition Info

Calories: 177

Total Fat: 14g

Carbohydrates: 7g

Fiber: 7g

Protein: 11g

Low Carb Gluten Free Cranberry Bread

A perfect low carb cranberry bread free from gluten, with fresh cranberries. This sugar-free bread uses the combination of stevia sweeteners and erythritol.

Prep Time 10 minutes

Cook Time 1 hour 15 minutes

Total Time 1 hour 25 minutes

Servings 12 people

Ingredients

- ❖ 1 1/2 teaspoons baking powder
- ❖ 1/2 teaspoon baking soda
- ❖ 1 teaspoon salt
- ❖ 2 cups almond flour
- ❖ 1/2 cup coconut milk
- ❖ 1 bag cranberries 12 ounces
- ❖ 1/2 cup powdered erythritol or Swerve,
- ❖ 1/2 teaspoon Steviva stevia powder

- 4 tbspoons unsalted butter melted (or coconut oil)
- 1 tspoon blackstrap molasses optional (for brown sugar flavor)
- 4 large eggs at room temperature

Instructions

- Preheat the oven to 350 degrees; grease and set aside a 9-by-5 "loaf pan.
- Whisk flour, erythritol, baking powder, stevia, baking soda, and salt together in a large bowl; set aside;
- Combine butter, eggs, molasses, and coconut milk in a medium sized bowl.
- Mix dry into wet mixture until well mixed.
- Fold in cranberries. Pour batter into ready-made pan.
- Bake, about 1 hour and 15 minutes, until a toothpick inserted in the loaf center comes clean.

- ❖ Transfer the casserole to a wire rack; let the bread cool for 15 minutes before removing the pan.

Nutrition Info

Calories 179 Calories from Fat 135

Total Fat 15g 23%

Saturated Fat 4g 20%

Cholesterol 72mg 24%

Sodium 276mg 12%

Potassium 38mg 1%

Total Carbohydrates 7g 2%

Dietary Fiber 2g 8%

Sugars 1g

Protein 6.4g 13%

Low Carb Focaccia Bread

It is also easy to make low carb focaccia bread as a garlic bread. Make sure you shaped the focaccia before baking to be flat and cut small slices through the dough halfway through. It makes it all cook evenly.

Prep Time: 15 mins

Cook Time: 30 mins

Total Time: 45 mins

Servings: 4 Loaf

Ingredients

- ❖ 2 tsp baking powder
- ❖ 1 tsp salt
- ❖ 4 eggs - medium
- ❖ 50 g coconut flour
- ❖ 5 tbsp psyllium husk
- ❖ 250 ml boiling water

Instructions

- ❖ Place the coconut flour, husks of psyllium, baking powder and salt in a large mixing bowl, then whisk until mixed.
- ❖ Add the eggs and blend. The mixture is going to be a very strong' play-dough' like consistency so at this stage don't work it too hard.
- ❖ Add a cup of boiling water and mix until well combined.
- ❖ Shape into a form of focaccia and put it on a baking tray lined with baking paper. Create diagonal cuttings through the dough using a sharp knife, sprinkle with plenty of salt, rosemary and put olives on top of the dough.
- ❖ Bake for 25-30 minutes, at 180C. When the center is no longer' spongy,' it is cooked.
- ❖ Serve cold with cheese, hot with butter, slices of avocado, onions, labna etc.

❖ Add plenty of flavors such as rosemary, garlic, salt etc.* Psyllium husk 100 percent fiber and once applied to water, swell and thicken to ensure you prevent any' eggy' taste. Used to thicken foods, this product is applied to gluten-free baking where it binds moisture and helps make breads less crumbly, and as a laxative. When taking psyllium, always drink plenty of fluids as the husks swell and absorb liquids from your stomach as it transits around.

Nutrition Info

Calories 528 Calories from Fat 234

Total Fat 26g 40%

Total Carbohydrates 58g 19%

Dietary Fiber 42g 168%

Sugars 5.9g

Protein 31g 62%

Cinnamon Raisin Swirl Bread

A low carb Cinnamon Raisin Swirl Bread which does the original good! For your holiday brunch or breakfast, enjoy this naturally sweet and wholesome treat.

Prep Time 20 mins

Cook Time 1 hr 10 mins

Total Time 1 hr 30 mins

Servings: 1 loaf

Ingredients

Filling:

- 1 tbsp Swerve Sweetener
- 1 tsp ground cinnamon

Bread:

- 1 tbsp baking powder
- 1/2 tsp ground cinnamon
- 1/4 tsp salt

- 1/2 cup coconut flour
- 1/2 cup almond flour
- 6 tbsp psyllium husk powder
- 1/4 cup California raisins chopped fine
- 2 tbsp Swerve Sweetener
- 2 cups egg whites (liquid egg whites work well but you can also measure out whites from regular eggs. It will be 8 to 12 whites, depending on the size)
- 4 tbsp melted butter divided
- 2 tbsp apple cider vinegar
- 3/4 cup hot water (almost boiling)

Instructions

- Preheat the/an oven to 350F, grease a loaf pan of 9x5 inches. Grease 2 large parchment paper pieces.
- Whisk the sweetener and cinnamon together in a small bowl. Set aside.
- Whisk the coconut meal, almond meal, psyllium husk powder, chopped raisins,

sweetener, baking powder, cinnamon and salt together in a large bowl.

❖ Add the egg whites, 3 tbsp of the melted butter, and vinegar with apple cider. Stir to mix. Slowly stir in hot water until expanding the dough.

❖ Turn the dough onto one of the grated parchment pieces and pat into a raw rectangle. Top with other parchment bits and roll out to about 8x12 inches. Brush and sprinkle with cinnamon filling with about half of the remaining melted butter. Tightly roll up and place seam-side-down in the prepared loaf pan.

❖ Brush with the rest of the butter. Bake until golden brown and firm to the touch for 60 to 70 minutes. Remove foil from oven and tent. Let cool down in the pan (this helps to keep it from deflating). Move to a cutting board or a serving plate once it cools.

Nutrition Info

Calories 132 Calories from Fat 59

Total Fat 6.58g 10%

Saturated Fat 3.27g 16%

Cholesterol 10mg 3%

Sodium 283mg 12%

Total Carbohydrates 12.36g 4%

Dietary Fiber 6.02g 24%

Protein 6.28g 13%

Jenni Treesong

Keto Low Carb Buns with Psyllium Husk

Very delicious low carb buns that taste just like bread with multigrain!

Prep Time 10 minutes

Cook Time 30 minutes

Total Time 40 minutes

Servings buns

Ingredients

- ❖ 4 tbsp boiling water

Dry Ingredients

- ❖ 1 tsp black sesame seeds
- ❖ 1 tsp white sesame seeds
- ❖ 2 tsp sunflower seeds
- ❖ 100 g blanched almond flour (about/around 3/4 cup tightly packed)
- ❖ 2 tablesp psyllium husk powder
- ❖ 1 tsp baking powder

- ❖ 1 tsp black chia seeds
- ❖ 1/2 tsp Himalayan salt
- ❖ 1/2 tsp garlic powder

Wet Ingredients

- ❖ 1 tabspoon apple cider vinegar (or lemon juice, white vinegar)
- ❖ 1 egg
- ❖ 2 egg whites
- ❖ 3 tabsp melted refined coconut oil (or butter, lard, shortening, ghee)

Instructions

- ❖ Oven preheat to 180C/350F.
- ❖ In a bowl, mix with a whisk the dry ingredients. Mix the wet ingredients in a separate bowl. Put those wet ingredients into the dry ingredients and apply a silicone spatula to blend.

- ❖ Pour in the boiling water gradually and start to blend. The dough is going to be fairly dense and expand as it absorbs water.
- ❖ Separate the dough into 5 balls and use your hands to shape 5 balls (the batter is sticky). You should rub some olive oil on your hands so the dough doesn't stick to you.
- ❖ Place the balls on a baking tray over parchment paper, and bake for 30 minutes. Take it out and let it cool or you'll burn your fingers before serving! These end up coming out piping hot!

Notes

- ❖ You can't substitute the psyllium husk powder.
- ❖ Do not leave the boiling water out please. Activate the psyllium you need it.
- ❖ Making sure to use REFINED coconut oil and not the usual extra virgin kind as you will get a gigantic taste of coconut.

- ❖ You may need to add 1-2 tablespoon of hot water to the batter, if you double the recipe.
- ❖ All our ovens are different, so if you find yours too cold, just add 5 more minutes in the oven, or cook them for 30 minutes at 190C/375F instead.

Nutrition Info

Calories 236 Calories from Fat 187

Total Fat 20.81g 32%

Saturated Fat 8.37g 42%

Cholesterol 42mg 14%

Sodium 41mg 2%

Total Carbohydrates 8.34g 3%

Dietary Fiber 5.34g 21%

Sugars 0.96g

Protein 7.53g 15%

3 Ingredient Paleo Naan (Indian bread)

Prep Time: 5 minutes

Serving: 6 small naans

Ingredients

- ❖ 1 cup coconut milk, full fat (canned)
- ❖ ½ cup almond flour
- ❖ ½ cup tapioca flour or arrowroot flour
- ❖ Salt, adjust to taste, optional
- ❖ Ghee (slather that bread!), optional

Instructions

- ❖ Preheat a crepe pan over medium heat, or nonstick oven.
- ❖ In a bowl, combine all the ingredients together, and pour ¼ cup of the batter over the pan.
- ❖ Turn/flip it over to cook the other side after the batter fluffs up and looks firm / mostly cooked (be patient, this takes a little time!).

- ❖ Serve immediately/straight away or cool on a wire rack.

Notes.

Options for Size:

- ❖ If your naan is a little sticky in the centre, you can put it on a baking sheet and bake at 350F for 5 minutes, or at 400F for a crispier flatbread for 10-15 minutes.
- ❖ If you wish to make a dessert crepe, pour in the batter and spread it as thinly as possible.
- ❖ If you don't use a non-stick pan, you'll need to use some kind of oil / ghee / fat to avoid the batter sticking. I have that carbon steel crepe pan and I love it.
- ❖ If your canned coconut milk has solidified the sugar, blend well before using.

Nutrition Info

Calories Per Serving: 129

15% Total Fat 9.6g

0% Cholesterol 0mg

0% Sodium 6mg

4% Total Carbohydrate 11g

Sugars 1.4g

2% Protein 1g

Ultimate Dairy-Free Keto Bread

Prep Time 5 minutes

Cook Time 30 minutes

Servings 4

Ingredients

- ❖ 1 oz. coconut flour
- ❖ 1/2 tsp. baking powder
- ❖ 1/4 tsp. salt
- ❖ 2 ounce. macadamia butter
- ❖ 2 large eggs
- ❖ 1 large egg white
- ❖ 1/2 tsp. erythritol
- ❖ 1/2 tbsp. psyllium husks powder

Instructions

- ❖ Oven preheat to 180 ° C (350 ° F). Layer a parchment paper sheet baking pan.
- ❖ Add/Combine all the dry ingredients in a small bowl, leaving out only the powder of

psyllium husks. The coconut flour is best sifted.

- Make butter with macadamia if you have none. Actually pulse the nuts in a S-blade food processor bowl (scraping the bowl sides once or twice) until you get runny oil.
- Mix in a medium bowl, using an electric mixer, the eggs and egg white. Add the butter with the macadamia and stir until well incorporated.
- Combine the mixture of eggs and dry mixture, then mix well. Add the psyllium husks powder at the very end, and mix a few more. If you find that the mixture runny, add coconut flour in another T and mix well.
- Use your hands or a spoon on the baking pan to shape four disks. To make this step less sticky, wet your hands.
- Bake within 30 minutes.

Nutrition Info

170 Calories, Net Carbs: 2.6 g, Protein: 6.5 g, Fat: 13.4 g (of which Saturated: 3.4 g, MUFA's: 9.3 g), Total Carbs: 7.5 g, Fiber: 4.9 g,

Jenni Treesong

Best Keto Bread Recipe

Prep Time 10 mins

Cook Time 1 hr 5 mins

Total Time 1 hr 15 min

Servings: 10

Ingredients

- ❖ 1 teaspoon salt
- ❖ 2 teaspoons apple cider vinegar
- ❖ 1 1/4 cups (5 ounce/143g) almond flour
- ❖ 5 tbspoons psyllium husk*powder
- ❖ 2 tspoons baking powder
- ❖ 1 cup (8floz/225ml) boiling water
- ❖ 3 egg whites
- ❖ 2 tablespoons sesame seeds, optional

Instructions

- ❖ Preheat the oven to 180 ° C (350 ° F), then butter and layer a 9x5 inch loaf tin with parchment paper. Set aside.

- ❖ The almond flour, baking powder, psyllium husk, and salt are mixed in a large bowl.
- ❖ Add the egg whites and the apple cider vinegar to the dry ingredients at medium speed with an electric mixer until a paste-like dough is formed.
- ❖ Stream in boiling water whilst mixing at low speed. Adjust the speed to high and mix for about 30 seconds, or until the mixture shapes the dough and the elastic play-dough. Watch out not to over-mix!
- ❖ Move the dough to the baking tin prepared, and smooth the rim. Sprinkle on the sesame seeds, lastly.
- ❖ Bake the bread for 55 minutes - 65 minutes or until the top is rising and puffing up like a traditional loaf of sandwich.
- ❖ Remove the bread from the oven then allow to cool slightly before being moved to a refrigerating rack.

- ❖ Refreshed slice once and enjoy! 2 Days to store the covered bread at room temperature. After 2 days I recommend that you put it in the refrigerator for no more than 2 more days.

Recipe Notes

If you can't find psyllium husk for some reason, you can add ground flax or linden meal.

Nutrition Info

Calories 53 Calories from Fat 27

Total Fat 3g 5%

Sodium 55mg 2%

Potassium 37mg 1%

Total Carbohydrates 4g 1%

Dietary Fiber 6g 24%

Protein 2g 4%

Keto + Low Carb Cornbread Muffins

This muffins are fully corn-free but without the high carb count they are reminiscent of real cornbread muffins. They're great as a side, snack or breakfast!

Prep Time: 15 minutes

Cook Time: 25 minutes

Total Time: 40 minutes

Servings: 12

Ingredients

- ❖ 1/2 cup unsweetened coconut milk (from a carton, not a jar)
- ❖ 5 tbsp salted butter, melted
- ❖ 1/4 cup (30g) almond meal
- ❖ 3 tbsp (27g) Swerve Confectioners
- ❖ 3 oz cream cheese, softened
- ❖ 1 cup (128g) coconut flour
- ❖ 3 eggs, slightly beaten
- ❖ 1/2 cup heavy whipping cream

- ❖ 1 1/2 tsp baking powder
- ❖ 1/8 tsp salt

Instructions

- ❖ Preheat the oven to 350 F.
- ❖ You don't need to grease the pan if you're using a silicone muffin pan, like I do. Nevertheless, if you don't use silicone, I would recommend that you grease it lightly or use liners for easy removal.
- ❖ Combine the eggs, heavy whipping cream, coconut milk, melted butter (slightly cooled), and cream cheese in a large bowl. Mix it up until the cream cheese is well-incorporated using a hand mixer. (It's all right, if you've got a few small flecks left.) Set aside.
- ❖ Combine coconut flour, almond meal, Swerve Confectioner, baking powder and salt in a medium-sized dish. Mix carefully.
- ❖ Using your hand mixer to add dry ingredients to wet, and mix thoroughly.

- ❖ Distribute the batter evenly across the holes, with the back of a spoon pressing the batter down a bit. (The batter is thick and the pockets are easily formed.) They are about 80 percent full.
- ❖ Put in the oven and bake for 20-25 minutes until the edges start to brown, and mostly clean the inserted toothpick. Don't overbow. Once you take the pan out of the oven, the middle should still be slightly soft (but not uncooked)
- ❖ Sweet, and have fun!

Nutrition Info

Calories 169 Calories from Fat 126

Total Fat 14g 22%

Saturated Fat 8g 40%

Cholesterol 64mg 21%

Sodium 105mg 4%

Potassium 105mg 3%

Total Carbohydrates 7.8g 3%

Dietary Fiber 3.7g 15%

Sugars 0g

Protein 4g 8%

Keto Flax Seed Bread

Prep Time 5 minutes

Cook Time 2 minutes

Total Time 7 minutes

Servings 2 Slices

Ingredients

- 1 tablespoon Softened Butter
- 4 tablespoons Organic Ground Flaxseed Meal
- 1 Large Egg
- ½ teaspoon Baking Powder
- ½ teaspoon Salt

Instructions

- Take your square Pyrex glass dish and add the butter. Melt for a few seconds in the microwave.
- Crack the egg into the bowl, and blend well with a fork.

- ❖ In a separate bowl, mix the ground flax seed, salt and baking powder, and blend.
- ❖ Adding all mixed dry ingredients, ground flax, salt, and baking powder to the baking dish and thoroughly blend all ingredients.
- ❖ It will turn into a dense layer. To ensure even cooking, flatten out the surface of the mixture.
- ❖ Two minutes in the microwave to cook.
- ❖ Until taking out, leave to cool for a few minutes.
- ❖ Use a spatula and pull the bread gently off the side of the platter. It should come out without any trouble after you turn it upside down.
- ❖ Take your knife and cut it half way to make two slices

3 Minute Low Carb Biscuits

Prep Time: 2 minutes

Cook Time: 3 minutes

Total Time: 5 minutes

Servings: 1 Servings

Calories: 392kcal

Ingredients

- 1/4 cup Cheddar Cheese
- 1/8 tsp garlic powder
- 1/8 tsp Onion powder
- 1/8 tsp Dried Parsley
- 1 tbsp Butter
- 2 tbsp Coconut flour
- 1 large Egg
- 1 tbsp Heavy Whipping Cream
- 2 tbsp Water
- 1/8 tsp Pink Himalayan Salt
- 1/8 tsp black pepper

- ❖ 1/4 tsp Baking powder

Instructions

- ❖ Melt butter for 20 seconds in a caffee mug by microwaving.
- ❖ Add the flour with coconut, baking powder and seasonings. Combine with a fork to add.
- ❖ Add the heavy whipping cream, egg, and cheese. Mix until blend.
- ❖ Microwave for three minutes. Remove from mug immediately and allow to cool down for 2 minutes.
- ❖ Slice, and have fun.

Nutrition Info

Calories: 392kcal, Carbohydrates: 9g, Protein: 15g, Fat: 32g, Fiber: 5g

Coconut Flour Psyllium Husk Bread - Paleo

Are you looking to have an easy low carb keto Paleo bread? Try this recipe for gluten-free psyllium bread in coconut flour. Breakfast or dinner is a tasty bread to serve.

Prep Time 5 minutes

Cook Time 55 minutes

Total Time 1 hour

Servings 15 slices

Calories 127kcal

Ingredients

- ❖ 6 tablespoons whole psyllium husks 27g, may want to finely grind
- ❖ 3/4 cup warm water
- ❖ 1 cup coconut flour 125g
- ❖ 1 1/2 teaspoons baking soda
- ❖ 3/4 teaspoon sea salt

- ❖ 1 pint egg whites 2 cups (or use 8 whole eggs)
- ❖ 2 large eggs
- ❖ 1/2 cup olive oil
- ❖ 1/4 cup coconut oil melted

Instructions

- ❖ Preheat oven to 350 degrees F.
- ❖ If not to use silicone pan, grease pan or line pan with parchment paper. I used that 8x4-in pan.
- ❖ Dump all ingredients and pulse until well mixed into a food processor. If you don't have a food processor you can use an electric mixer mixing cup.
- ❖ Spread batter into loaf pan with 8x4. Smooth top.
- ❖ Bake for 45-55 minutes or until brown edges are inserted and clean the toothpick.
- ❖ Let the bread sit for 15 minutes in a saucepan. Remove the bread from the saucepan and allow the rack to cool.

Notes

Original recipe used an egg carton that may give rise to an odor of ammonia. The recipe has therefore changed to 1 pint egg whites and 2 whole eggs.

Nutrition Info

Calories 127 Calories from Fat 120

Total Fat 13.3g 20%

Sodium 243mg 10%

Total Carbohydrates 6g 2%

Dietary Fiber 4.1g 16%

Protein 3g 6%

Homemade Nut and Seed Paleo Bread

Prep Time: 10 min

Cook Time: 40 min

Total Time: 50 minutes

Serving: 12 -15 slices

Ingredients

- 1/4 cup chia meal (just blender or grind chia seed in a coffee grinder) or use ground flaxseed
- Pumpkin seed for topping and Extra poppyseed
- 1/2 teasp sea salt
- dash of black pepper
- Optional 1 teasp spice mix of choice (garlic, rosemary, Italian, etc.).
- 1 – 2 teasp poppyseed (plus extra for topping)
- 1 1/4 cup almond flour
- 5 eggs (6 if you want more fluffy)
- 1/3 cup coconut oil or avocado oil

- ❖ 1 teasp white vinegar or apple cider vinegar
- ❖ 3 to 4 tablesp tapioca flour (if you are using more egg, add 4 tbsp).
- ❖ 1/2 tsp baking soda

Instructions

- ❖ Preheat oven until 350. Grease a parchment paper pan or line of 9 x 5 breadpan. Set aside. Use an 8⁄4 pan for higher higher bread.
- ❖ Whisk your eggs, butter, and vinegar in a small saucepan.
- ❖ Combine the flours, poppyzeed and seasonings in another tub.
- ❖ Attach your wet ingredients and blend well to dry ingredients.
- ❖ Pour batter into greased pan and cover with additional and poppyseed pumpkin seeds.
- ❖ Covered Bake for 20 minutes. Then uncover and continue baking for 15-20 more or golden and clean knife in the center.

- ❖ Depending on your oven, should all be about 35-45 minutes together. If you used 8 x 4 or baked higher, you may need to bake longer.
- ❖ Clear from the frying pan and let cool.
- ❖ Wrap, slice and store the paleo bread in foil or plastic wrap. Keeps well in refrigerator for up to seven days or freezer for up to three months.

Notes

If you're looking for a vegan or egg-free option you can try to replace the eggs with 3/4 cup aquafaba. It bakes but not much rises. All yummy!

Low Carb Pumpkin Bread

Prep Time: 15 minutes

Cook Time: 45 minutes

Total Time: 1 hour

Serving: 20

Ingredients

- 15 oz. can of pumpkin puree
- 2 cups granulated of sugar substitute
- 3 teaspoons of baking powder
- 2 teaspoon vanilla extract
- 3 tablespoons of pumpkin pie spice
- 3 tablespoons of cinnamon powder
- 1/4 teaspoon sea salt
- 10 large eggs
- 3 cups of almond flour
- 1 cup of golden flax meal
- Optional
- Cream Cheese Frosting
- 8 oz package of softened cream cheese

- ❖ 4 tablespoons of heavy whipping cream
- ❖ 1 cup of sugar-free confectioners sugar

Instructions

- ❖ Preheat the oven to 350 ° C.
- ❖ Grease two loaf pans 8x4 inches well.
- ❖ Beat the pumpkin puree, sugar substitute, and vanilla extract with an electric mixer until it is well blended.
- ❖ Then add one at a time in the eggs to make sure that they beat before completely combined.
- ❖ Add the almond flour and flax seed, baking powder, spices and salt to the wet batter.
- ❖ Remember batter is going to be thick Pour the batter into the two pans and bake for 45 minutes at 350 degrees, or until an inserted toothpick comes out clean.

Notes

This recipe makes two large loaves of low carb pumpkin bread and froze well.

Nutrition Info

Calories: 200 Total Fat: 15.8g Saturated Fat: 5.5g Cholesterol: 59mg Sodium: 60mg Carbohydrates: 4.8g Fiber: 2.9g Sugar: 0.8g Protein: 6.4g

Jenni Treesong

Cheesy Skillet Bread

Easy low carb skillet bread with a sumptuous cheddar cheese crust. This recipe for keto bread is good for soups and stews, and makes the BEST low carb Thanksgiving stuffing!

Prep Time 10 mins

Cook Time 16 mins

Total Time 26 mins

Servings: 10

Ingredients

- ❖ 1 tbsp butter for the skillet
- ❖ 2 cups almond flour
- ❖ 1/2 cup flax seed meal
- ❖ 2 tsp baking powder
- ❖ 1/2 tsp salt
- ❖ 1 1/2 cps shredded Cheddar cheese divided
- ❖ 3 large eggs lightly beaen
- ❖ 1/2 cup butter melted

- 3/4 cup almond milk

Instructions

- Oven preheat to 425F. Fill a 10-inch oven-proof skillet with 1 tbsp of butter and put in the oven.
- Whisk the almond flour, flax seed meal, baking powder, salt and 1 cup shredded cheddar cheese together in a large bowl.
- Adding the eggs, melted butter, and almond milk until well combined.
- Remove the hot skillet from the oven (remember to put the mitts on your pan), and swirl the butter to the side of the brush.
- Pour batter into a casserole and smooth the top. Sprinkle with 1/2 cup remaining cheddar.
- Bake for 16 minutes to 20 minutes, or until browned around the edges and set midway through. Cheese should be well browned up on top.
- Remove, then allow it to cool for 15 minutes.

Recipe Notes

Serves 10. Each serving has 7.2 g of carbs & 4 g of fiber. Total NET CARBS = 3.2 g.

Nutrition Info

Calories 357 Calories from Fat 276

Total Fat 30.63g 47%

Total Carbohydrates 7.9g 3%

Dietary Fiber 4.77g 19%

Protein 12.48g 25%

Turmeric Cauliflower Buns

This 4-Ingredient Turmeric Cauliflower Buns are an easy side dish that is grain-free, low-carb and super healthy.

Prep Time: 30 mins

Cook Time: 30 mins

Serving: 6

Ingredients

- ❖ 2 eggs
- ❖ 2 tablespoons coconut flour
- ❖ 1 medium head of cauliflower
- ❖ ¼ teaspoon ground turmeric
- ❖ pinch each of salt and pepper

Instructions

- ❖ Oven preheat to 400 ° F.
- ❖ Line a parchment-papered baking sheet and set aside.

❖ Take your cauliflower and cut off the base with a sharp knife. Use your hands to split the cauliflower into florets and pick off any green parts. Give quick rinse and pat dry to the florets.

❖ Next, make cauliflower rice by putting the florets with the "S" blade in a food processor's bowl. Pulse until the cauliflower is about or almost the size of the rice for about 30 seconds. You should have about two cups of cauliflower rice that is firmly packed.

❖ Layer the cauliflower rice with around a teaspoon of water in a microwave-safe cup. Cover with plastic wrap then poke a couple of holes to let the steam run away. Microwave around 3 minutes of the cauliflower rice. Instead, the cauliflower rice can be steamed in a steamer basket on the stovetop.

❖ Uncover the bowl and allow about 5 minutes to cool the cauliflower rice. Then put the cauliflower rice in a nut milk bag or a clean

- dish towel with a large spoon. Extra moisture squeeze out, be careful not to burn your palms.
- ❖ In a small mixing bowl, add the cauliflower rice and stir in the eggs, turmeric and a pinch of salt and black pepper.
- ❖ Use your hands to shape the blend into 6 buns and put them on the baking sheet.
- ❖ Bake for 25-30 minutes, or until slightly browning on top.
- ❖ The cauliflower buns are best served directly from the oven, soft. They don't cool or heat well (they're going to get mushy), but they're so delicious that you're going to eat them immediately!

Nutrition Info

Calories Per Serving: 59

% Daily Value

3% Total Fat 2.1g

21% Cholesterol 62mg

6% Sodium 151.7mg

2% Total Carbohydrate 6.6g

Sugars 2.4g

9% Protein 4.5g

2% Vitamin A 26.7μg

79% Vitamin C 47.2mg

3% Calcium 31.2mg

4% Magnesium 17mg

Buttery Low Carb Flatbread

The best from the sliced bread. Mostly because it is gluten-free, fried and in butter slathered.

Prep time 5 mins

Cook time 2 mins

Total time 7 mins

Serves: 4

Ingredients

- ❖ 1 tbsp Oil for frying
- ❖ 1 tbsp melted Butter-for slathering
- ❖ 1 cup Almond Flour
- ❖ 2 tbsp Coconut Flour
- ❖ 2 tsp Xanthan Gum
- ❖ ½ tsp Baking Powder
- ❖ ½ tsp Falk Salt + more to garnish
- ❖ 1 Whole Egg + 1 Egg White
- ❖ 1 tbsp Water

Instructions

- ❖ Whisk the dry ingredients together (flours, xanthan gum, baking powder, salt) until well blended.
- ❖ Add the white egg and egg and gently beat for incorporation into the flour. The dough is about to start forming.
- ❖ Attach the tablespoon of water and start working the dough to allow the moisture to absorb the flour and xanthan gum.
- ❖ Cut the dough into 4 (four) equal parts and press out each segment with a fastener.
- ❖ Heat over medium heat a large skillet, and add oil.
- ❖ Fry each flat-bread on each side for about 1 min.
- ❖ Sprinkle with butter (when warm) and garnish with salt and chopped parsley.
- ❖ Just split the dough into 5 balls instead of 4, if you want a smaller portion!

Nutrition Info

Serving size: 1 flatbread Calories: 232 Fat: 19 Carbohydrates: 9 Fiber: 5 Protein: 9

Jenni Treesong

Paleo Gluten-Free Low Carb English Muffin

A paleo low carb English muffin recipe which is soft and buttery inside, crusty on the outside. This gluten-free English muffins are easy to make with 5 ingredients in 2 minutes!

Prep Time 2 minutes

Cook Time 3 minutes

Total Time 5 minutes

Ingredients

- ❖ 1 pinch Sea salt
- ❖ 1/2 tsp Gluten-free baking powder
- ❖ 1 large Egg (or equivalent egg whites)
- ❖ 3 tbsp Blanched almond flour
- ❖ 1/2 tbsp Coconut flour
- ❖ 1 tablesp Butter (or ghee, or coconut oil)

Instructions

- ❖ Melt ghee (or butter) in a ramekin or other container that is safe for microwaves or ovens, about 4 in (10 cm) diameter with a flat base. It takes about 30 seconds to do so. (If you only use an oven, melt it in the oven while it is preheating. Remove once melted.) Adding the remaining ingredients and stir until well mixed. Let sit for a minute, to thicken the mixture.

- ❖ Microwave Method: Microwave until firm for about 90 seconds.

- ❖ Oven method: Bake at 350 degrees F (177 degrees C) for about 15 minutes, until the top is firm and spring-y to the touch.

- ❖ Travel along the edge of a knife and flip over a plate to release. In the toaster, slice in half, then toast.

Recipe Notes

If you want more / smaller slices, instead of a ramekin, you can as well make it in a mug, and just pop those in the toaster in batch.

Serving size: 2 large slices (entire recipe)

Nutrition Info

Calories 307

Fat 27g

Protein 12g

Total Carbs 8g

Net Carbs 4g

Fiber 4g

Sugar 2g

Cauliflower Tortillas

Great low carb alternative to traditional flour tortillas or corn.

Prep Time 30 minutes

Cook Time 20 minutes

Total Time 50 minutes

Servings 6 tortillas

Calories 37

Ingredients

- ❖ 1/2 medium lime, juiced and zested
- ❖ salt & pepper, to taste
- ❖ 1/4 cup chopped fresh cilantro
- ❖ 3/4 large head cauliflower
- ❖ 2 large eggs

Instructions

- ❖ Preheat an/the oven to 375 degrees F., and line the baking sheet with parchment paper.

- ❖ Trim the cauliflower, cut it into small size, uniform pieces and pulse in batches in a food processor until you get a consistency similar to a couscous. The finely riced cauliflower should be packed into about 2 cups.
- ❖ Place the coliflower for 2 minutes in a microwave-safe bowl and microwave, then stir again and microwave for another 2 minutes. If you're not using a microwave, then a steamer works just as well. Put the cauliflower in a fine cheesecloth or thin dishtowel, squeeze out as much liquid as possible, making sure you don't burn. Gloves are suggested for dishwashing, as it is very hot.
- ❖ Whisk the eggs into a medium bowl. Add cauliflower, coriander, lime, salt and pepper to taste. Blend well until combined. Use your hands on the parchment paper to shape 6 small "tortillas"
- ❖ Bake for 10 minutes, flip each tortilla carefully, and then return to the oven for

another 5 minutes to 7 minutes or until completely set. Place tortillas on a wire rack to slightly cool off.

❖ Heat on a medium sized skillet. Place a baked tortilla into the oven, slightly press down and brown on each side for 1 to 2 minutes. Repeat with tortillas left on.

Keto Fiber Bread Rolls Recipe

These Low Carb and Keto Fiber Bread Rolls Recipe are made perfectly and are extremely delicious and irresistible to make. One look at them will persuade you to try and get them right at this moment.

Prep Time 10 minutes

Cook Time 40 minutes

Total Time 50 minutes

Serving: 11 Serving Size: 1

Ingredients

- 15g (3Tbsp)Psyllium Husk
- 250g (1 Cup)Greek Yogurt
- 4 Eggs
- 150g (1.5 Cups) Almond Flour
- 30g (1/4 Cup) Protein
- 1 Pkt (16g)(4tsp) Baking Powder
- 75g (3/4 Cup)Potato or Oat Fiber
- 4 Tbsp (25g) Oil

- ❖ 2 Tbsp Water
- ❖ 2 Tbsp Vinegar
- ❖ 1 tsp salt

Instructions

- ❖ Heat the oven until 150C or 300F.
- ❖ Blend dry ingredients together.
- ❖ Separate eggs, and first mix all the egg whites. Deposit aside.
- ❖ Mix well, the egg yolks.
- ❖ Stir in yogurt and all the wet ingredients.
- ❖ Keep adding all the combined dry ingredients spoon by spoon.
- ❖ Add egg whites at the end and gently and blend properly.
- ❖ Cover the bowl for half an hour, and let it rest.
- ❖ Prepare a sheet of Parchment paper for baking.
- ❖ When relaxed, make small balls with wet side, which you then flatten with hands to create rolls a bit at the end.

- ❖ Once everything is on the baking sheet, add a bit of Potato or Oat Fiber to obtain the white look after baking.
- ❖ With your super Kaiser Roll Shaper Gadget knife, press each Roll to give it the perfect finishing touch.
- ❖ Place/Put in the oven and bake 40 Minutes.
- ❖ Bon Appetit.

Notes. Notes.

You can use Potato Fiber or Oat Fiber for this recipe to achieve the results which are the same.

Nutrition Info

Calories: 177

Total Fat: 14g

Carbohydrates: 7g

Fiber: 7g

Protein: 11g

CONCLUSION

The keto diet is a flexible and fun way to lose weight, with plenty of delicious food options.

Before plunging into a Ketogenic diet you should always check with your doctor. Completing a blood panel is also a very good idea, just as you would before doing a steroid cycle. This is not your usual diet, where you cut off your daily intake a small amount of fat and lose a few pounds. The world's top experts use ketogenic dieting to maintain amazing shape-and can be used by you too - as long as you carefully diet which supplement.

Printed in the USA
CPSIA information can be obtained
at www.ICGtesting.com
LVHW012157140524
780323LV00033B/1003